PREFACE BY DR. SUSAN VELDA

Tinnitus is a phenomenon of our time. On the other hand, it was already here before and troubled a lot of ordinary people as well as more famous ones. Many Tinnitus sufferers have been met with lack of understanding, not only by his closest of family and friends, but often even by doctors. This can lead to isolation, worsening of the subjective perception of tinnitus and thus, depression.

It affects almost all ages, from early adolescents to seniors. Etiology differs. Tinnitus is often caused by multiple contributing factors: organic and/or functional. Yet, the result is always the same: unpleasant subjective perception of tone or noise, which can significantly interfere with normal life, relationships and work activities.

If tinnitus does not have an organic basis, which should be solved in a radical way, there is a solution. This solution, which Peter describes in detail, has helped thousands of patients return to normal life. You just need to do something for yourself, have strong will, and stay focused on your goal and the result will come.

Dr. Susan Velda
Senior ENT Medical Specialist

INTRODUCTION

"If I could cure my tinnitus, why not you? Yes, it is possible. I am living proof."

Peter Studenik MS

A few years ago, I went through the same painful journey as you or your loved one. In time, I successfully cured my tinnitus and hyperacusis, when every day sounds, seem louder than they should. Since then, I had helped many tinnitus sufferers with their treatment in personal consultations, over the phone, via Skype or by email. As time went on, more and more people asked me for help. I provided this help for free after work. One day, I was asked by larger group of tinnitus sufferers to contribute regularly to their internet forum. This was a challenge for me, as on the one hand, I felt the need to help others; on the other, I did not have any free time. I decided it would be best to stop providing help. In my heart, however, I struggled as I knew there was no one else who could help them and inspire them. Therefore, I started looking for a way to help those who needed it while at the same time allowing me to have enough free time.

One day my friend asked me, "Why don't you write a book where you will share your story, knowledge and answer frequently asked questions?" My first reaction was that it sounded like nonsense, as I had never written a book before. But over time, I began to see that it was possible, and after a great deal of effort, I wrote this book. The first release in 2013 was written in Slovak, then, in 2016, the Czech language, and in 2017, I had my book translated into English. The first part of this book is about my

story; I describe what I went through. The main reason for this is to give people inspiration and hope that their tinnitus can be cured. The second part contains information about all the steps I took to cure my tinnitus. The third part contains answers to frequently asked questions. This part is new to this sixth edition. I have added the answers and have provided advice for those questions most commonly asked. I also publish new findings regularly on my website:
www.icuredmytinnitus.com.

    I know that tinnitus can be cured. The fact that you are holding this book means that you are on the right path to healing. The only thing that is required is to stay on your take action plan and persevere. So, once again I keep my fingers crossed for you and want to stress that tinnitus and hyperacusis can be healed. I am living proof.

Peter Studenik MS

SIX-STEP THERAPY

"Start by doing what's necessary; then do what's possible; and suddenly you are doing the impossible."

Francis of Assisi

I suffered from tinnitus for four years and today I hear silence again.

My tinnitus started after a loud concert in 2009 and was perceived as a constant whistling and ringing in my ears. At that time, I couldn't concentrate on anything or even sleep. I heard it all days and nights long and I was very afraid. After two weeks, I was in such a panic that I forced myself to go to an ENT specialist. He performed a lot of tests and confirmed that I had tinnitus and hyperacusis. He prescribed me drugs to stop acute tinnitus. But it didn't help at all. After three months of unsuccessful treatment, the doctor said, "You have chronic tinnitus, learn how to live with it." My life collapsed at that moment.

As I couldn't live with tinnitus, I didn't give up and tried everything to stop it. I visited many other specialists - neurologists, homeopaths, Chinese medicine specialists, nutritionists, body movement specialists, etc. Unfortunately, none of them helped me and I felt more and more helpless.

After three years of troubles, I started to look at tinnitus from a broader perspective and found out that tinnitus was being investigated by Pawel J. Jastreboff, Ph.D., Sc.D., Professor at Department of Otolaryngology at Yale University.

I immediately read all his research, understood what tinnitus is, how it starts and why standard treatment fails. I got in touch with him and he confirmed that my tinnitus could be cured. I started to believe that I could cure my tinnitus, and together we found the way. At the same time, I started therapy with a psychologist to restore psychic balance and well-being. After nine months my tinnitus stopped.

Following my cure, I noticed how much my personal and working life had changed. I realized, that very important step in curing my tinnitus was finding and resolving all the causes including the long-term stress, work overload, anxiety, and relationship problems.

Today I clearly see that my cure was combination of multiple aspects, which can be divided into these three parts:

- **Physical** - exclude physiological cause with ENT specialist/neurologist, physiotherapy to fix the cervical spine and jaws, diet change, exercise and sinusitis clean.
- **Sound therapy** - understanding how tinnitus starts and disconnect your fixation of the brain on tinnitus, utilizing special sound.
- **Psychical** – obtain stress and emotional relief, resolving long term stress, setup proper work-life balance.

I have not had tinnitus since 2013. The therapy for tinnitus that I underwent is equally effective for all types of chronic tinnitus. It doesn't matter if your tinnitus was caused by a loud sound, ear inflammation, surgery, injury, hearing damage, etc., the chances are the same. It does not matter which sounds you hear, whether it is a whistling, ringing, buzzing, roaring, clicking or any other sounds. I don't even notice tinnitus now, neither in times of silence, nor at night.

To cure my tinnitus, all these steps were important. I was very consistent, committed and proactive in each step. All steps needed to be done correctly and precisely. Sometimes it was not easy, but as I saw that my tinnitus was decreasing, it gave me the inner strength to continue.

Six-steps which helped to cure my tinnitus:

1. Exclude objective cause.

It could be an ear infection, sinusitis infection, spin problem, etc. This must be investigated by Medical Specialists before taking any further steps.

2. Understand the real cause and mechanism of chronic tinnitus and that it can be cured.

This was discovered by Pawel J. Jastreboff, Ph.D., ScD. His scientific model is described in detail in the next chapters. In this step I also describe my story, so you can understand better, how my tinnitus was cured and why standard treatment fails.

3. Sound therapy plus daily tinnitus measurement

Sound therapy is done with pink noise. It disconnects fixation of our brain on tinnitus. The sound therapy noise can be generated either by noise generators, such as Siemens, Phonak or Audifon), or, for example, a hifi mp3 player such as Fiio MK3 combined with Sennheiser MX 365 headphones). Please find actual available devices on my web (devices article):
www.icuredmytinnitus.com

Daily tinnitus measurement.
Even if it seems that the volume of tinnitus is the same every day, it is, in fact, changing a little bit, based on many factors. As you measure your tinnitus every day, you will find that the volume of your tinnitus is changing, maybe very small changes, but changing. And it's very important to measure these changes by sound therapy devices.

Tinnitus diary.
As tinnitus is changing, you will be able to determine what is increasing/decreasing your tinnitus. This helped me very much during my cure.

4. Emotional and stress relief.

Find the way how to work with your emotions and express them (e.g., many men don't cry and many women don't express anger), how to manage long-term stress, how to avoid pressure in work and personal life, how to solve anxiety and excessive self-observation of any medical concern, how to fix relationships with your partner or parents. After most of the emotional releases, my tinnitus volume became lower.

5. Fix the spine and jaws.
Body postures at work, during sleeping/eating, sports or some other activities can increase your tinnitus. If so, you will need to unblock spine and jaws, etc., in cooperation with a physiotherapist.

6. Diet change.
Many meals and drinks make your tinnitus louder. Find out which ones.

Find and solve broader consequences based on findings in tinnitus diary.

Important note:
During my cure I measured my tinnitus every day (described in the chapter *Tinnitus volume measurement* and noted it in my tinnitus diary. With daily measurements noted in my tinnitus diary, I found out which items from steps (meals, drinks, situations, and persons) worsen my tinnitus and needed to be fixed. Also, I saw how my tinnitus was decreasing in time. You can download my tinnitus diary and pink noise which I used during my cure, here for free on my web:
www.icuredmytinnitus.com

STEP ONE

EXCLUDE OBJECTIVE CAUSES AND STANDARD THERAPY WHICH HELPS.

EXLUDE OBJECTIVE CAUSE

This is essential before any further steps. Please visit your medical specialists to exclude physiological cause such as ear infection, etc. It is mostly done by ENT specialists and neurologists. They may decide to recommend you visit next specialists, such as dentists, physiotherapists etc. Please undergo all examinations and therapies which were recommended by your medical specialists. Even if physiological cause is a very rare reason, you need to do this first.

From standard treatment utilising a hyperbaric chamber, this can and does help some people. So, I recommend trying it. In my opinion, and from my experience, you would need to have this treatment 20 times. Ask your medical specialist about this treatment.

DRUGS

I only used antihistamine anti-vertigo medication (broadly used to cure tinnitus) in the beginning for a few months and ginkgo supplements. None of this helped me and as I wrote, I completely dropped the drugs. I also did not take any medication to help me to sleep.

"Opposing Opinion" from Michaela N.:
"The worst at the beginning of chronic tinnitus can be disturbed sleep. In this situation, many unfortunate people can come up with sleeping pills that are addictive. Twenty years ago, the chief of neuroscience at the hospital in Prague recommended me the addictive anxiety reducing drugs to be a common long treatment for tinnitus. I took it and got addicted! I would therefore like to warn everyone about these "side effects". Doctors often think that tinnitus is worse than addiction, which is not right. The addictive preparations are a trap - they work very well in the short term, but if the addiction develops, the benefits are just zeroed, and that's the way to hell."

If you need sleeping or calming pills, ask for last generation ones. First generations can make your tinnitus worse. Also, this is only a temporary solution.

In the next chapters, you will understand my story, what I underwent, what helped me and what did not helped me. You may save a lot of your time, to avoid things that didn't help and focus on items which lead to your cure.

STEP TWO

UNDERSTANDING THAT TINNITUS CAN BE CURED,
HOW IT STARTS AND WHAT TO ADRESS TO GET
COMPLETE TINNITUS.

MY STORY AND HOW IT STARTED

"The biggest mistake is to make tinnitus patients believe there is nothing we can do"

Dr. Pawel Jastreboff
professor, Yale University of medicine

It was a Saturday evening 2009. Cypress Hill, a well-known hip-hop band, which I used to listen as teenager, came to a music club in Prague. I went with two friends. The atmosphere was great. We arrived before the concert started, had a few beers and were looking forward to the band we had listened to a lot as teenagers. The opening band started playing. They were good and we listened to it from the balcony. Later we came down to the stage for Cypress Hill. The volume increased significantly. I had a feeling that it was much too loud but assumed that the promoters knew what a right and secure volume level was. Since no one else was complaining, I decided to relax and began to enjoy the atmosphere of the performance. Cypress Hill was amazing. They played all the hits I knew. We were jumping around for two hours. When the music stopped, everything seemed fine; I was completely relaxed, happy, and deafened. After the concert ended, I jumped on a tram, came home, and lay down in bed. I was still deafened, in the same way as I had experienced many times before, afterparties. I was not worried, as it had always passed the next day, so I fell asleep happy and completely exhausted.

THE FIRST DAYS

"Feelings of helplessness, immobility, and freezing. If hyperarousal is the nervous system's accelerator, a sense of overwhelming helplessness is its brake. The helplessness that is experienced at such times is not the ordinary sense of helplessness that can affect anyone from time to time. It is the sense of being collapsed, immobilised, and utterly helpless. It is not a perception, belief, or a trick of the imagination. It is real."

Dr. Peter A. Levine

The next morning, I woke up, showered, got dressed, brushed my teeth and did other routine activities. But something was different – I was still very deafened. I grabbed some chewing gum, hoping it will help, popped some in my mouth (like it helps on an airplane flight) and I went to work. In the beginning, I could ignore it, but as the day passed, I gradually noticed it more and more. I had never experienced this before and was starting to get nervous. That first night, I fell asleep, frightened. The next day was the same and the fear slowly turned into panic. My hearing was as if I was underwater. I constantly asked people to repeat themselves, because their words were not clear. I could not eat, I felt only fear. I knew I had screwed up my hearing. I could not sleep at night, and for the first time I said this to my wife. All night I was looking out the window at the dark, and could not sleep. I started to hear the whistle in my ears, but what most bothered me at that time was that I was not able to hear properly.

On the third morning, I woke up and finally, my hearing was ok. I was happy. I brushed my teeth, sang, dressed up and went to work. Along the way I turned on the radio, but I could not stand the music, as it was very "sharp" (high frequencies hurt), so I quickly turned it off. When I arrived at work, everything seemed perfectly fine. At noon, I went to the canteen for lunch.

Once I entered the canteen, I could not stand the sound of forks and knives. It was unbearable. During the whole lunch, I suffered intensely; every sound hurt my ears. I just wanted to eat quickly and return to silence. I came back to the office and finally found peace.

I continued to experience the same phenomenon for several days and it was getting worse. And, if that wasn't bad enough, the occasional whistling in my ears that had started after the concert became constant, with no let up, day or night. It was so intense it kept me from sleeping. All night long I was experiencing great fear. The worst thing during this period for me was that I could not sleep properly, because of the never-ending whistling. I realised that if I could not sleep well, my job performance would be bad, and I would be restless and irritable. And this was exactly what happened. My work performance suffered – I was either apathetic or anxious. The same was happening at home. Either I was arguing with my wife, or I became completely detached and did not listen–to what she said. It was similar at my business, which I operated, in addition to my full-time day job – a Pizza restaurant. I soon realised that if I didn't resolve the problem of tinnitus, I would lose everything. And as you will see later in the book, this is exactly what happened.

Because almost every sound hurt, I started wearing earplugs. The earplugs made sounds less sharp. On one hand it was a relief, but on the other hand, whenever I had used ear plugs, I perceived whistling even more.

Roughly, a week later, I started conducting internet research on my symptoms, to find a diagnosis that would result in an action plan to end my problem. Based on my symptoms, I quickly realized that I had tinnitus. This discovery triggered even greater panic, as everything I read from both doctors and tinnitus sufferers indicated that tinnitus cannot be cured. Apparently, I would have tinnitus for the rest of my life!

Someone recommended that I watch a documentary about the famous Czech guitar player Michal Pavlicek, who suffered from tinnitus for many years. It had taken my last hope – if he could not cure his tinnitus, as rich and famous as he was, how could I? And I discovered that he was not the only famous musician suffering from tinnitus: Bono Vox, Barbara Streisand, Eric Clapton, and many others also had it. These were rich and famous people who I believed had tried everything to get rid of tinnitus, and even they could not heal it. I started to feel despair.

After I read all the painful stories, I said to myself: "I cannot live like this." I must do everything to be completely cured (not only partially). Because life with tinnitus made no sense to me. I must find the way.

"Opposing Opinion" from Michael N.:
I disagree with Peter's conclusion that life with tinnitus does not have sense. I live 20 years with tinnitus, I can say that even though it sucks to live with it, I can handle it. I was supported by antidepressants drugs to stabilise my mood and to calm down. Based on recent discoveries I suggest a completely natural and non-addictive pill called Kava-Kava. I would avoid using addictive drugs. However, I recognised that if a person cannot sleep, it's really horror.

At that time, I read a huge number of articles and internet discussions and visited websites devoted to tinnitus. Unfortunately, none of these sources gave me hope that a cure was possible. Everything that I read focused on mitigation or masking techniques (such as having a fountain in one's bedroom), and the need to learn accept life with tinnitus.

All of this happened during a two-week period that seemed like years.

TREATMENT THAT DIDN'T HELP

Everywhere on the Internet, people wrote that it is important to start treatment as soon as possible. After two weeks, I was in such a panic that I forced myself to go to a medical specialist. He performed standard tests and confirmed that I had tinnitus and hyperacusis. I remember the awful feeling that came with his diagnosis. Based on reading Internet articles and discussions, I already knew that these conditions are forever. Apart from having tinnitus and hyperacusis, he confirmed I was totally "healthy". In my opinion, this is the worst combination: you suffer a lot and the doctor tells you that you are ok. He prescribed antihistamine anti-vertigo medication to increase blood flow to my ears. From the Internet, I knew about the possibility to take steroid infusions and so I asked him about this. He replied that I came too late. He said that those infusions only make sense within the first three days. I asked for other option which would help. He assured me that there is nothing else and that after treatment with antihistamine anti-vertigo medication, it will subside and eventually disappear. So, I believed him and started the antihistamine anti-vertigo medication treatment. I was a bit relaxed, and at the beginning I had the feeling that tinnitus decreased slightly. But as time went on, I noticed that the whistling remained equally unbearable. Due to hyperacusis I started to use earplugs everywhere and they made the tinnitus even worse. I had no idea that was possible, as the doctor did not warn me. I saw other doctors, hoping for alternative treatments, but they also prescribed antihistamine anti-vertigo medication. So, I took antihistamine anti-vertigo medication, with the hope that the whistling would disappear. But it did not disappear at all and my conditions got worse and I fell into great despair.

CHRONIC TINNITUS

After 3 months of unsuccessful treatment, the doctor said "You have it for life, it is chronic. Now it is too late to start with any other treatment. Learn to live with it."

To which, I replied, "What???!!!!"

I was totally speechless, I did not ask him how this was possible when he assured me that antihistamine anti-vertigo medication would help, which other treatments he meant, or why he initially claimed that there is no other treatment.

I felt like I was robbed of my last hope. I knew that I could not live like this. "That's not a life," I thought, "I will never learn to live with tinnitus."

I came home completely devastated, my work performance deteriorated, my marriage began to disintegrate. I stopped communicating with the co-founder of my pizza business. I was depressed. I lost weight because I didn't eat. In every spare moment, I focused on whether the whistling was strong or weak that day. A few times I experienced false hope: a couple of days I thought that the whistling was getting better, but later it reverted to the previous level. I was completely desperate, and I started to give up on treatment and on life in general. Moreover, every sound caused me great pain, so I wore earplugs everywhere. I began to avoid people and increasingly closed into myself. I completely distanced myself from my neighbors, family, and friends. I just went to work and then came directly home. I tried to go into the woods and be at peace with myself, being surrounded with nature, but unbearable whistling accompanied me everywhere. I would never hear the "silence of the forest" again. This remained the same for several months, I was constantly sleepy, exhausted and terribly frightened. And I felt tremendous anger towards myself.

In my head, I interrogated myself intensely:

"Why did I have to go to that concert?"
"Why I did not use earplugs?"
"Why, did I believe that antihistamine anti-vertigo medication would help?"
"Why didn't I go to the doctor the next day and have an steroids infusion?"

What's more, I hated the whole music production team at Prague Music Bar and Cypress Hill, because the volume at the concert was far too high.

ALTERNATIVE TREATMENT

"Complicated health problem needs at minimum three specialists."

Chinese proverb

After several months on antihistamine anti-vertigo medication, I decided to quit taking this, and stopped visiting doctors because it became clear to me that the doctors did not know how to help me. Having seen that traditional medicine would not heal my condition, I decided to give alternative medicine a try. I began seeing a Chinese doctor, changed my diet, drank awful tasting tea, underwent acupuncture, attempted to "unblock" my spine, and started an exercise routine. I also started taking different supplements to increase blood flow, such as gingko. Unfortunately, none of these things helped. Alternative therapy gave me hope back, but when I tried everything and nothing helped, I fell back into complete despair.

At the time, I was arguing everyday with my wife, boss and business partner. All around me, my life was crumbling, but I was not able to do anything about it. And it did not matter to me. All I wanted was to get rid of my tinnitus. Nothing else in the world existed for me. I slowly fell into a state of apathy. I still occasionally sought help via the Internet or tried something new. But these were only sporadic attempts and slowly I began to surrender and admit that I screwed up my life and there was no way out.

FIRST HOPE

After some time of inactivity and complete apathy I realised that I absolutely could not live like this and I invested my last energy to find real treatment. So, I began to search the entire Internet again and identify opportunities for further treatment, mostly from abroad. I found many websites that promised to cure tinnitus. I paid and tried several methods, but nothing worked. These treatments were always based on the assumption there is something wrong in the ear and the aim of the proscribed exercises, pills or diet was to improve blood flow to the ear. As all were built on the same flawed principle, none of them worked.

After a few months of constant searching, I found a page that treated tinnitus differently. In the beginning I was skeptical, but they wanted no registration and no money. This increased my confidence a little, so I began to read the page. Within a few days, I read all the content on the website. I was excited. Finally, something new and different! I read the website multiple times. Everything that I read gave me confidence and I felt that this was something that could really help. The website was founded by a neurologist, which boosted my confidence even more. So, I regained hope and looked forward to trying that method. The website was www.tinnitus-pjj.com.

BEGINNING OF REAL CURE

Reading this web site of Pawel Jastreboff, I realised what tinnitus really is and what it is not. This understanding was the first step in the treatment of my tinnitus.

All that I learned on this page made sense, although at the beginning I was very skeptical. After trying countless other treatments, I had trouble believing that something could help. Every doctor that I visited claimed that tinnitus was a lifelong condition, that nothing could be done, and I needed to accept it. I read the same thing on all the discussions on the Internet. There were so many desperate people and no help.

The only hope at that time was what I read on this website. After I read the website a few times and I felt that I understood, I immediately contacted the founder of this method Dr. Jastreboff with many questions. He responded to all my questions in several e-mails and calmed me down. I knew that this method made sense and so I began looking for someone in the Czech Republic or the Slovak Republic who knew this method and used it.

At that time, there were just two doctors in the Czech Republic who were familiar with this method. I was lucky that one doctor was in Prague, where I lived. I immediately contacted her. The second doctor was from east part of Czech Republic (in a faraway part of the Czech Republic). Nobody else in the Czech Republic knew about this method. Today TRT therapy is better known and I believe that in the future more doctors will become familiar with it.

After contacting the doctor in Prague, I waited roughly a month and half until she had time to see me. I was looking forward for real cure. I expected that everything would be different, but when I walked into the waiting room desperation overcame me.

Again, white space, again waiting in the waiting room. I felt like I was back in the standard doctors waiting room, and he would conduct a standard examination and, in the end, would not be able to help me. But I was there, so I underwent the examination. The examination was like the previous ones, so my sense of desperation increased. After the standard "ORL" examination, I passed the examination of the volume of tinnitus in a soundproof room. I thought to myself, "At least this is something different from all of previous the examinations." My tinnitus loudness was very low, as was expected at around 5 db. Even though the volume of my tinnitus is objectively very low, it was extremely uncomfortable to me. I already knew this from the Internet. Subjectively, I perceived the tinnitus as very strong, like all who suffered from it. But the next minutes were different. The doctor explained to me the nature of tinnitus and how even when the volume of tinnitus is very low, I feel it like a horrible sound. Everything she told me I already knew from the website, but it was amazing to hear it from a real doctor.

My diagnosis, as before: chronic tinnitus with hyperacusis. But this time it was not labelled "untreatable." Instead, the doctor assured me that this treatment would work and that there was recently a young girl who, under her care, had been treated successfully. It sounded like a miracle to me. She told me to avoid silence **and to use earplugs in the normal environment. I protested the use of earplugs and we agreed that I would use only half-sized earplugs.**

The doctor also gave me the following:
- A booklet from Siemens (which manufactures special handsets priced at approximately $1,100. Fortunately, you will not need them).
- Record of "pink noise" – pink because I also had hyperacusis (this is explained later in the book).
- Instructions on how to use pink noise, how long to listen to it and at what volume.

She also suggested psychosomatic therapy. I refused initially, asserting that I did not need it.

The next day I began my treatment, which is called "Tinnitus Retraining Therapy" or "TRT".

These are the instructions I received:
- Read the booklet, to understand what tinnitus really is. This point I could skip because I had read about tinnitus from the site www.tinnitus.org and www.tinnitus-pjj.com. You can read it in the second part of this book.
- Listen to pink noise. The doctor offered me a special device from Siemens, but I did not want them. First, the price was $1,100 and secondly, it looked exactly like the devices for half-deaf people. Instead, I decided that I would listen to the noise from high-quality MP3 player with quality headphones, which I already had. The booklet from Siemens discouraged the use of an MP3 player, (but only because they were afraid that with MP3 player, people will not listen to it long enough - 8 hours).
- Once again, I was asked to consider the offer of psychotherapy. From her point of view, it was very beneficial for tinnitus sufferers.

In the evening, I copied the pink noise from the CD into the computer as a WAV file. It is important to have sound without compression (such as MP3). It must not be compressed, as MP3, because the conversion makes changes in character of sound. I uploaded file to MP3 player and set it to repeat. In the morning when I woke up and everything was quiet, I adjusted the volume of noise according to the instructions from the doctor. It is important that the volume of the noise is lower than the volume of one's tinnitus. Tinnitus noise must be always louder than the pink or white noise. Otherwise, it is not TRT, but so-called "camouflage." I set it for each ear separately because my tinnitus was louder in my right ear. I put on the headphones and went to work. I should have listened tinnitus 8 hours a day. I managed it this way:

I got up at 7:00 AM, I immediately started to listen to the noise and listened to it while I got dressed, bathed and all the way on the commute to work at 9:00 AM, for a total of 2 hours. I would leave work at 5:30 PM and then put on the earphones and listen to the noise until I went to bed at 11:30 PM, for an additional 6 hours. So altogether, I managed to reach the required time of 8 hours per day.

When listening to the noise, I did all the usual activities, traveling, eating, and watching television. The sound is so quiet that you feel as if you have headphones in their ears, but the player is turned off. Your brain is perceiving pink noise, even if you do not hear it.

One of the arguments why to buy a special noise generator from Siemens was that with headphones you cannot easily reach the required listening time of 8 hours per day. However, in my case it was possible and for me it was much more comfortable – and **free.** If you use headphones in public transport nobody will look at you. Many people can even use them at work.

Over time I have changed my opinion on noise generation devices. This is because other companies started to offer noise generator devices such as Audiofon, which are much cheaper and almost invisible. However, if you have a good mp3 player and good earphones, it is enough.

And I listened pink noise every day. I did not miss a single day and after a few weeks I started to feel relief. My brain calmed down. I still heard tinnitus, but I was not so annoying. I knew that this treatment worked and started to believe that I just needed to continue, and I could live without tinnitus.

During the first months, I felt relaxed during the time when I was hearing the pink noise. When I turned MP3 player off, my tinnitus reoccurred, and my body was again in stress. For me the pink noise was amazing, because at least there were a few moments when I felt relief.

I continued with TRT therapy for a few months and I was getting better. I increasingly believed that this method would completely cure me, and I would live without tinnitus. Also, I decided to accept the recommendation to undergo psychotherapy. It helped me to reveal things associated with tinnitus. Gradually, as I resolved those issues which were found during psychotherapy and continued with TRT therapy, I ceased to perceive tinnitus. One day after six months of treatment, I was totally without tinnitus. It has been quite common, that I did not perceive tinnitus with MP3 player on and hearing the pink noise. But that day was different. I had my headphones on for 8 hours, the required amount time of day, so I turned my MP3 player off. I discovered that it was already off, because the battery had died. For first time, I did not perceive tinnitus without the MP3 player on! I was very happy, and it confirmed that the method was working. I was not completely cured, but I knew that if I followed through with my treatment, I would heal my tinnitus completely.

For the next six months, I continued to listen to the noise and undergo psychosomatic therapy. Slowly life began to return to normal. My hyperacusis also disappeared. However, I admit that the next six months I was not as consistent. It often happened that I did not charge the player or had other reasons for not listening to the pink noise as recommended. Next half year, I continued treatment, even though I was cured. It is recommended to continue treatment for six months after the symptoms disappear, to prevent the return of tinnitus, but I was confident that I did not need to continue treatment. More important, to prevent tinnitus is to resolve your psychosomatic and social consequences. When it these issues are addressed, tinnitus will disappear forever.

All these years later, I do not hear tinnitus at all. Thanks to psychosomatic therapy, I changed my life quite radically for the better. This was a significant element of my healing. I am back to my normal life and even much better than before my tinnitus began.

I have also made some changes to my habits. For example, nowadays when I go to a party, the theater or a concert, or anywhere else where sounds are very loud, I bring earplugs. In my opinion, everyone should do this to prevent tinnitus.

I underestimated and misjudged the value of psychosomatic therapy. It ended up being a very important part of my treatment. The first reason was that everything collapsed around me and I could not deal with it alone. The second reason was that we found a psychosomatic reason for my tinnitus and solved it. Again, from my point of view, it is very important to enrich TRT therapy with psychological and psychosomatic work. I believe that the psychotherapy and psychological contexts resolved the root causes of my tinnitus. You will find more detail in the next chapters ahead.

"Opposing Opinion" from Martin K.
What really helped me was hypnotherapy. I undergo self-hypnosis based on MP3 records that affect the subconscious perception of tinnitus sounds. On the web, you can find an expert to help it prepare for you.

HOW TINNITUS STARTS

Importance of hearing

Sound has great importance for monitoring of our environment. Animal's hearing, which live in constant fear of their lives because of attacks from predators, must be very sensitive. The ability of animals to develop extremely acute hearing, by which they could detect the very small sounds of an attacker a long way off, contributes to the survival of that animal. Sound warning signals produce acute anxiety, prompting appropriate action to avoid attack, or to attack. This is called survival reflex. We respond in the same way to the sound of a car horn, by automatically and urgently and immediately looking for the potential danger. Some sounds can be identified as warning signals, while others can evoke a feeling of security or pleasure. We have this experience every day with sounds that alarm us, or sounds that soothe us such as music, or the sounds of nature. Many sounds naturally evoke strong emotions of one sort or another.

How we hear

The conscious awareness of sound is located near the surface of the brain, when a pattern of electrical activity goes from hearing nerve and reaches the part of the brain - auditory cortex. The hearing nerve has about 30,000 fibers, and patterns of electrical activity in these fibers are matched with other patterns, which are held in the auditory, or hearing memory. The inner ear, which changes sound waves into these electrical patterns, is a surprisingly noisy place. This continuous mechanical and electrical activity in 17,000 hair cells can be monitored with sensitive, computer enhanced, listening devices. This noise is called otoacoustic emissions. Most of what we hear is a sequence of different sounds, like speech or music. In infancy, new sound experiences are stored in an information hungry, but relatively empty auditory cortex. Later, there is a continuous process of matching familiar memory patterns with those coming from the ear.

Each time a pattern from the ears is matched with a pattern in the auditory memory we have the experience of hearing and recognising a sound. Putting together these matched patterns starts a process of evaluation. Another part of the brain close to this initial hearing center is involved in the meaning of what we hear, and in interpreting the language. If it's a foreign language, we can hear the sound, but we may not understand the meaning.

Meaning of sounds

When a sound has special or critical meaning, like the baby waking at night, or the creaking of a floorboard, or the sound of our first name, we respond to it in an automatic manner, even if the volume is very soft. This happens after a short learning period, and the responses can remain just as strong during our whole life. During sleep, the conscious part of the brain is 'shut down' so we don't hear, see or feel anything. However, the mother still wakes to the baby stirring even though she has just slept through a thunderstorm. What could wake the baby. This shows that weak patterns of sound, if they have great significance and meaning, can be detected by subconscious pathways or filters, between ear and part of the brain - auditory cortex, even during sleep. These filters can enhance and amplify important sounds, and at the same time, suppress or habituate sounds of no interest.

Conditioned responses

Conditioned responses trigger activity outside the auditory system. There are large numbers of connections with the limbic system which is concerned with emotion and learning. It also stimulates the autonomic nervous system which activates the body, to prepare for any eventuality. In situations of danger, or perceived threat, the familiar 'fight or flight' response is triggered.

This involves high levels of autonomic function; tense muscles, raised heart and breathing rates, sweating - complete opposite to the state of relaxation. They rightly preclude sleep, or concentration on other, less important tasks. Limbic and autonomic responses to things we always dislike, involve the same mechanisms, but are less strong, and are called aversive conditioned responses. A universal aversive response occurs with the sound of nails scraping across a piece of glass. Every sound that we hear and learn the meaning of, has an "emotional label" attached to it, which may change from time to time according to how we feel, and the context in which we hear it. For example, the sound of the next-door television set may be either acceptable, or unpleasant and intrusive, depending on whether it belongs either to a well-loved friend or relation, or a neighbor which we don't like.

Tinnitus sounds

In 1953 Heller and Bergman performed a simple experiment. They placed 80 tinnitus free individuals (university members) in a sound proofed room for 5 minutes each, asking them to report on any sounds that might be heard. The subjects thought they might be undergoing a hearing test, but in fact they experienced 5 minutes of total silence. 93% reported hearing buzzing, pulsing, whistling sounds in the head or ears identical to those reported by tinnitus sufferers. This simple experiment shows almost anyone can detect background electrical activity, which is present in every living nerve cell in the hearing pathways as a sound. Although some areas of the auditory system may be more active than others, every neuron will contribute to some extent to the final perception of tinnitus. These electrical signals are not evidence of damage, but compensatory activity that occurs all the time in the auditory system of each one of us. Compensation can occur as a response to changes in our sound environment (e.g. silence), to hearing loss, which a natural part of ageing may be, or to exposure to sudden noise. It's good to think of the sounds produced by this compensatory activity as 'the music of the brain'. Of those who experience persistent tinnitus, population studies have shown that about 85% do not find it intrusive, disturbing or anxiety provoking, which something tinnitus sufferers find very hard to believe. The reason for this is not so much because of the quality or loudness of the tinnitus is different. In fact, it was found that tinnitus is of a very similar type of sound in those who are bothered by it and those who are not.

The main difference is that those who find tinnitus troublesome, evaluate and perceive it as a threat, or an annoyance. Volume is same. Tinnitus may also emerge for the first time when something else unpleasant or frightening is happening to us. In these situations, tinnitus is classified as a warning signal, relating either to a bad experience, or to negative thoughts about its meaning or outcome. Just as an animal is alerted to danger by the sound of a predator, and focuses solely on that sound to survive, so those who consider that tinnitus is a threat or warning signal are unable to do anything but listen to it. It is part of the mechanism that all animals have developed for self-preservation, although clearly in this situation it is not working to our advantage. Many people complain of the loss of silence, something they previously greatly treasured and enjoyed, before tinnitus became persistent. Tinnitus becomes part of the bereavement for this loss.

What happens, even in mild cases of persistent tinnitus, is that a conditioned response/reaction is set up to the tinnitus sound. As the conditioned response is part of the subconscious brain, and automatic, what you may be thinking about tinnitus at any time, is irrelevant to the reaction produced. Moreover, it is the reaction to tinnitus, which is creating distress, not the tinnitus itself - another difficult concept for some. The degree to which unpleasant feelings about tinnitus (from the limbic system) and increased tension (from autonomic system stimulation) are experienced, dictates the severity of the tinnitus. The loudness and quality of the sound heard, is irrelevant.

Tinnitus as a something new
When tinnitus first emerges, it is a new signal. There are no

memory patterns, and no means of categorizing it. Any new experience produces an 'orienting response' where we are forced to pay attention until the signal is classified and understood. Until proper evaluation has been undertaken of what tinnitus means, it will be regarded with understandable suspicion. Many 'sufferers' only experience mild annoyance from tinnitus because of this orienting response, but it may be sufficient to promote the need to seek help. A typical, and reasonable anxiety is 'will it get worse?' or 'what happens if it goes on forever?'

When tinnitus becomes a threat

For many sufferers, tinnitus is quite threatening. Some people fear that tinnitus means they have serious illness. Others are convinced that the experience of 'disco tinnitus' means permanent damage to the ear, rather than the temporary protective changes by the brain., which are normal and universal. There are patients who worry about the possibility that tinnitus means they have a brain tumor, blood clot, or some serious mental illness. Many people fear that tinnitus will get louder, continue forever, and cannot be cured. The concept that tinnitus is invading one's 'right to silence' constitutes a threat, very like the territorial invasions that all animals experience. It is often feared that tinnitus will continue to spoil peace and quiet, interfere with concentration at work, quiet recreational activity and the ability to sleep at night.

Incorrect advice

Unfortunately, these fears may be enhanced by professional advice, or reports from other sufferers, who have had a bad reaction to tinnitus. Many doctors and other professionals still advise patients that there is nothing that can be done about tinnitus, and that it will go on forever. Other people fear that tinnitus may mean that their hearing is becoming impaired. Tinnitus may be the consequence of a mild age-related hearing impairment, rather than the other way around. It is still only twice as common in hearing impairment, as in normal hearing. In any event, the threatening qualities of the tinnitus are enhanced by beliefs and negative ideas about tinnitus or associations that have been formed, not any physical changes that may or may not have occurred. Finally, many tinnitus sufferers are angry about the treatment, or lack of treatment, or inappropriate advice that they have received. They may feel guilty for having submitted to treatment, which they think, is the cause of their tinnitus. Fear, anger and guilt are very powerful emotions, which are intended to enhance survival-style, conditioned reflex activity, and consequently these emotions greatly increase attention on the tinnitus. In our experience, tinnitus improves when the patient overcomes these feelings and stops dwelling on thoughts of injustice.

Fear and tinnitus

For some patients, extreme fear of tinnitus results in a phobic state developing, very similar to that of the fear of spiders, frogs, small spaces, flying etc. Many tinnitus sufferers also have other phobias, suggesting common mechanisms at work. In the treatment of any phobia, a slow process of 'desensitization' must be used. First, you must confront the feared object, learn to experience it without reacting, and then to accept it as a normal phenomenon that does not, in any way threaten. Many aspects of tinnitus retraining are common to these techniques.

In other people, the response to tinnitus is milder, though still negative in its meaning. Annoyance and although strong emotions may not be evoked, the limbic and autonomic systems are still being stimulated to produce aversive and intrusive emotions which reduce life quality. Most importantly, these emotional responses ensure that tinnitus persists, rather than habituates naturally. These negative qualities of tinnitus, which make people seek help, are created outside the hearing mechanism, and therefore cannot be helped by a purely audiological, or the ear-related approach. This is the reason for the failure of tinnitus treatments, before TRT.

WHAT TINNITUS IS / WHAT IT ISN'T

Tinnitus is whistling, ringing, buzzing, roaring, clicking and other sounds that one perceives. My tinnitus was a high whistle like train breaks. The worst aspect for me was the nights when I could not sleep. Also, walking in the woods, was very uncomfortable, as I always enjoyed silence before, but whistling accompanied me – like everywhere else.

Whistling could be acute and chronic.

If you have had an ear infection or were at a noisy concert, played violin, shot a gun, had a firecracker explode near your ear, and you have later experienced whistling or any other sound in your ear, visit a doctor to confirm that everything is already all right (for example, an ear infection is cured, or any other physiological cause).

If you were at a concert, just visit your doctor and for few days completely avoid loud sounds while also avoiding complete silence. You may have acute tinnitus that will pass in a few days. During this time, it is good to have an open window at night to hear street sounds. If it is cold, a fountain or a humidifier will suffice.

If, after a few days, your acute tinnitus does not stop and you (and your doctor) have not found any physiological cause of your tinnitus, you likely have chronic tinnitus. And if your doctor confirmed that your tinnitus has gone into a chronic variant, this is the right book for you. I repeat once again, visit a doctor to exclude physiological cause. Do not worry too much, the number of people who have tinnitus due to physiological causes is very small.

So, if you have a diagnosis of chronic tinnitus without a physiological cause, as I did (and like most people who suffer from tinnitus), we can look at what chronic tinnitus is and what is not.

Well, let's start with what it is not. Since a doctor has confirmed that you are otherwise healthy, but you feel horrible, he probably will not help you. Chronic tinnitus is not a problem with the ear itself or with whistling in your ear, but with the perception of this sound by your brain.

This has come from Dr. Jastreboff, a neurologist who, because he is neurologist, was looking at the problem from a wider perspective and in doing so, has identified the real cause.

I will give a simple example of scientific research. As an experiment, healthy people were taken to a soundproof room. Scientists told those people that they will play sound and these people should seek to hear the sound. The result was that the majority of the people started to hear tinnitus, when they were focused on it. This means that it is the normal sound of a healthy body. The question is why tinnitus is bothersome for some and others do not even notice it.

The brain has the ability to filter the sounds it perceives. This is explained by a simple example to which everyone can relate. Imagine yourself in the midst of a noisy crowd as you might expect to find at a pub or busy office. In my case, my name is Peter. If someone calls the name "Thomas", I will not even register it and will continue with my activities - undisturbed. But if someone in the crowd calls my name, I always will hear that and turn my head automatically.

My trouble started when I was at a very loud concert, where my ears were damaged. It is best to imagine the forest through which a storm passes and strong wind damaged trees. I hurt my ears by damaging the hair cells (which are like trees in forest). But the body is tremendously self-healing, and so it began to work immediately on renewal, increasing cell activity in the ears to restore the original condition. This increased cell activity is accompanied by increased volume of normal sound and is known as acute tinnitus or "disco tinnitus". Acute or disco tinnitus usually lasts several hours or days, but three days is considered a critical limit. If, after about three days, acute tinnitus does not disappear, we will start to feel this sound as unpleasant. We start to fear it, to perceive it as dangerous. Well, as with any dangerous or important sound, your brain starts to amplify that sound. This is an ancient mechanism of our brain, which helped us to survive in the wild. The more we are afraid of it and the more we want to get rid of it, the stronger the tinnitus is. The more we try to get rid of it, the more desperate we become, because we eventually conclude that it cannot be cured. Certainly, you remember the terrible feeling you experienced when you first read about tinnitus on the Internet. And it is very likely that your tinnitus has become worse since visiting a doctor or reading Internet discussions. This is because the brain has begun to consider tinnitus an important or a dangerous sound and therefore decided to amplify it even more.

I followed all instructions from the doctors and tried everything possible. Nothing helped, though the doctors promised it would.

Often, after this phase, resignation and depression occurs and everything starts to fall apart. Man is misunderstood by others and falls into despair. I repeat, for all those who have tinnitus or those who knows people with tinnitus,

misunderstand tinnitus. I could not live life fully with tinnitus, nor enjoy anything. With tinnitus, I could only survive – the quality of life was miserable.

So, it is better to find your way to cure your tinnitus. Since you now know that chronic tinnitus is not a problem with your ear, but how your brain perceives and amplifies this sound, you know what to look for. The same thing occurred to the discoverers of TRT therapy. The discoverer of the real cause of tinnitus is Pawel

J. Jastreboff, PhD., Sc.D. He began to examine how it would be possible for the brain to cease to focus on tinnitus, the entirely natural sound that generates the activity of each person's cells.

He gradually found out that if the ears and the brains get different sensations, the perception of tinnitus is reduced. And if those with tinnitus perceive these different sensations for a long time, their tinnitus will disappear completely.

After years of research, he found that two sounds are appropriate. White noise and pink noise. These are sounds that play all the frequencies in equal volume. White noise plays the entire spectrum of sound, while pink noise has a cropped spectrum of high-pitched sounds. I used pink noise because I also suffered from hyperacusis. If you do not have hyperacusis you will use white noise. Both sounds can be compared to the sound of a waterfall that you can hear from a long distance away. This is a very pleasant sound; it can be described as a sweet or silky waterfall sound in the distance.

As noted earlier, the concept is illustrated with a simple example that everyone has experienced. Surely you have already been in a crowd of people in which someone calls another's name. The caller calls out the name loudly. Usually you do not even realize it. But if someone calls your name, whether or not you were the person intended, you will always be alerted and automatically turn around to see if you are being called. The brain will amplify the sound of your name to get your attention, and for you to react. So, as you can see, some sounds are amplified by the brain and some are reduced. And that's how it is with tinnitus in your ears. When your brain begins to perceive this sound as being dangerous or somehow important, it becomes chronic tinnitus. The longer you suffer from tinnitus, the more dangerous this sound will be perceived by the brain and the more it will increase continuously. In this phase you do not have a chance to cure by "ear treatment" because it is the natural sound of every healthy person – it is cell activity (but in your case just amplified). When I understood this, I realized why no drugs or massages, or infusions could help resolve my chronic tinnitus.

If you have chronic tinnitus, you need to focus on getting the brain to ignore the sound again. This is the way to take back the life you had before your tinnitus.

It is good to understand why your brain started amplifying the sound. After all, it was ignored for all your life. It can be triggered by noise, inflammation, spinal jam, or STRESS (therefore, psychotherapy could be an important part of your healing). It is an increased activity of the cells and therefore this natural sound is stronger in the beginning. As I mentioned before, it is called disco tinnitus. If one is lucky, their disco tinnitus goes away, and their life returns to normal. Those less fortunate will experience this sound after a few days as a problem and the brain fixates on it.

WHAT TO AVOID

Avoid complete silence. This is very important. Many people with tinnitus, which started by exposure to loud sounds such as music or a gunshot, naturally try to avoid sounds. But in silence you will feel tinnitus even more. So, save your earplug usage for very noisy environments such as parties, concerts, cinemas, the subway, etc. I suggest listening to some sound such as nice music. I have often listened to the sounds of nature, such as forest sounds, waterfalls, or whale's calls.

When there is significant silence, the brain is not at rest, but vice versa. In these situations, the brain is on guard. This is a paradox which I will explain. I will use an example from nature, where we all come from. Do you know when the greatest silence occurs in nature, when there is complete silence? In just one moment. When the predator approaches. Then all the animals will freeze and perceive every little, tiny sound. In addition, the brain strengthens all the sounds in this stress mode. So, when you are in complete silence, for example, at night with your windows closed, your brain is permanently on alert. In the past, there were no sound proof windows and we always heard some sounds outside. Even at night. birds, wind, rain, all this prevented complete silence. People in that time apparently did not even have a chance to perceive tinnitus. In English-speaking countries, this is called "sound enrichments".

Here are advices to avoid silence:
- If you have plastic windows, open them slightly to hear street sounds.
- Get a fountain in your home, put it in the living room and leave the bedroom door open at night.
- When you are at home, enjoy relaxing music, or the sounds of nature (such as the forest, sea, etc.).

- I enjoyed a lot of walks in the forest, where there are many sounds.
- Listen to the pink or white noise 8 hours per day, be consistent.

Go out in public, do not stay at home, tea houses and quieter cafes are ideal.

Talk about what bothers you, your friends, do not stay alone, friends could recommend you other great things.

Because tinnitus is stress-intensive, try psychotherapy, or psychosomatic help. Do not be alone with your problem. ASK for HELP. People are here to help you.

Avoid excessive noise. I guess that's obvious, but it's worth stressing. Excessive noise causes disco tinnitus. When you go to the cinema, your tinnitus will be louder for 1-2 days. Theoretically it does not matter at all, but it will psychologically knock you down. So, when you go to the cinema, bring your earplugs and take them out after the movie is finished. Please celebrate New Year's Eve without fireworks, avoid the shooting range, noisy concerts, and so on. For example, if you are a professional violinist, use the EtyPlugs, EPRO-ER, DLO earplugs. They are expensive, but they suppress all frequencies equally, so the sound you hear through them will not be distorted. Those are used by most of the world music stars and they know what they are doing. But use them only in noisy environments.

Those few simple recommendations will help you calm your nerves. You will be less stressed.

STEP FREE

SOUND TINNITUS RETRAINING THERAPY, SOUND DEVICES, PINK NOISE AND HOW TO DO IT RIGHT.

SOUND THERAPY

Successful tinnitus cure is a result of retraining, relearning and solving broader consequences. Once the tinnitus loses its sinister meaning, however loud it has been, or however unpleasant it may seem, it does begin to diminish, and in many cases, may not be heard ever again. In some cases, firmly held beliefs are hard to alter, particularly where there is a conviction that tinnitus is only related to ear damage which cannot be fixed. Retraining the subconscious auditory system to accept tinnitus as something that occurs naturally, does not spell a lifetime of torture and despair, and is not a threat or a warning signal. Retraining the subconscious auditory system can take some months and occasionally even years. You can follow my recommendations in this book or be guided by professionals with experience in this field. However, many people can be helped by understanding the Jastreboff model and applying the principles of retraining. For people who also have co-existing or pre-existing anxiety or depression, it can take longer to change their feelings about their tinnitus.

Retraining
Tinnitus Retraining Therapy is not simply an abstract learning exercise. In the subconscious part of the brain concerned with hearing, beyond the inner ear, but before conscious perception of sound takes place, subconscious filters, or networks of nerve cells are programmed to pick up signals on a 'need to hear' basis. Think again of the way we invariably detect the sound of our own name, or a distant car horn, or a new baby stirring in sleep, whereas we may be unaware of the sound of rain pounding on the roof or surf beating on a seashore. Retraining therapy involves reprogramming or resetting these networks which are selectively

picking up 'music of the brain' in the auditory system.

Tinnitus retraining first involves learning about what is causing the tinnitus. The result of this and other therapy including psychotherapy and sound therapy, the strength of the reaction against tinnitus gradually reduces. This reaction controls the setting of subconscious filters which are constantly looking for threats. With strong reactions, the filters are constantly monitoring tinnitus, but without a reaction, habituation occurs, as it does to every meaningless sound that is constantly present. Firstly, the disappearance of the reaction means that sufferers no longer feel bad, or distracted, and normal life activities can be resumed – sleep, recreation and work, as before. Secondly, as the auditory filters are no longer monitoring the tinnitus, it is heard less often and less loud. As a result, it can finally become a friend instead of an enemy.

Think, now, how much of this treatment depends on being able to believe that tinnitus results from normal compensatory changes in the hearing mechanism, rather than irreversible ear damage. While it is important to have a proper examination by an ear specialist, those professionals who themselves believe that tinnitus is an 'ear' phenomenon cannot help your tinnitus. Fortunately, few specialists have already an understanding based on the Jastreboff neurophysiological model (Jastreboff P.J. 1990).

Switching the tinnitus off

The presence of any continuous stimulus results in a process called habituation, whereby the individual responds less and less to the stimulus, as long as it does not have any special significance. Think of moving to a new house, from the quietness of the countryside, to live by a busy road. At first the traffic sounds are disliked and appear very loud. As this reaction diminishes with time - habituation of reaction, there is an automatic reduction in the perception of traffic sounds - habituation of perception. The final stage of habituation is when the signal is no longer detected, and cortical neurons are unresponsive.

With tinnitus, this means that it is no longer heard, or only on a very occasional basis. The important difference is that even when it is heard, it no longer produces any unpleasant feelings. In my case, it is not heard at all. As the goal is to get rid of tinnitus reaction, rather than tinnitus perception. Provided you have achieved this, then TRT is always successful, and permanent. It is important to distinguish between the role of the ear in the emergence of tinnitus (e.g. disco tinnitus, or the Heller and Bergman effect) and the persistence of tinnitus with an aversive response to it. Despite the importance of hearing change (temporary or permanent) in triggering an emergence of tinnitus, a recent study of tinnitus clinic patients showed there was no significant difference in hearing between the tinnitus group and normal population statistics.

Sound generators

Wearable sound generators (which look like hearing aids), or mp3 player with earphones have an important role. Tinnitus masking was at one time thought to be useful in that it simply made tinnitus inaudible. In fact, this proved to block tinnitus habituation, as it must be audible for habituation to occur. Habituation to any signal cannot occur in the absence of its perception. Imagine trying to habituate your response to spiders, which you hate, simply by avoiding them.

Much better long-term results can be obtained if wide band noise is used at low intensities while the tinnitus can be heard at the same time. Sound generators contain many frequencies, and therefore gently stimulate all the nerve cells in the auditory pathways allowing them to be more easily reprogrammed - increasing their plasticity. They must be fitted, and instruction given by a trained professional – since you are not a "trained Professional. You can either get a sound generator from a professional, or you may take my recommendations to use the mp3 and earphones. In my case I successfully used MP3 (Cowon D2) player with good headphones (YUIN PK2). Those are not available anymore, so check my web for devices which are available today here: www.icuredmytinnitus.com

Silence is bad

Emergence of tinnitus is often dependent on silence. Most tinnitus is first heard at night in a well soundproofed bedroom, or a quiet living room (Heller and Bergman 1953). Persistence of tinnitus depends not only on the meaning attached to it, but also to the contrast it creates with the auditory environment. Contrast contributes greatly to the intensity of any perception. Thus, a small candle in the corner of a large, darkened room seems to be dazzlingly bright, until the room lights are switched on making it virtually invisible. Everyone, especially tinnitus patients should avoid extreme silence, and retraining programmer will always use sound enrichment. Make sure there is always a pleasant, non-intrusive background sound - like a large slow fan, or an open window, and purchase a device for generating nature sounds. Smart phones can be used with a wide variety of 'apps' which produce nature sounds and white or pink noise. Choosing what sound is right for you may take some time. Nature sounds are always the best, as they are already habituated, and usually produce feeling of relaxation, calm and well-being. Avoid masking tinnitus, but have some sound present during day and night. Remember, filters are working 24 hours a day, even when asleep, and so, also should sound enrichment. Many tinnitus patients have decreased sound tolerance and for this reason often seek very quiet environments – see the Hyperacusis part in this book. They are their own worst enemy. In all cases, sound enrichment should be available, using pleasant sound sources, to break the silence. TRT is available in relatively few clinics, but the techniques are spreading and gradually being learned and used in an increasing number of ORL and audiology departments around the world.

TECHNICAL EQUIPMENT

When choosing a device, you have options (below, examples of what I have used in the past). These devices may no longer be available. However, I regularly monitor the availability of devices for sound therapy and regularly update recommended devices on my web here:

www.icuredmytinnitus.com

First option - high-end MP3 player and high-quality headphones. The price is around 120 USD (20 USD headphones, 100 USD MP3 player)

You need a quality MP3 player and headphones because it is important for the brain to hear all the frequencies well. Cheap headphones and MP3 players will not suffice, as they can play it only at normal volume (but you will listen at very low volume).

Be aware that the listening volume must be very low. So low, in fact, that it can only be played by high-quality headphones in conjunction with a high-quality MP3 player. I had the Yuin PK2 headphones and the COWON D2 MP3 player. You won't find Yuin headphones anymore but look at my web for available devices. I check and test them regularly and update here:

www.icuredmytinnitus.com

I strongly do not recommend using a smart phone, because:
- Number of volume level steps is 15 (mp3 players has 60-120) and you would not be able to see if your tinnitus is louder or weaker than day before (volume steps are too big to monitor difference).
- Sound therapy would be disrupted by messages and calls.

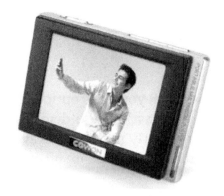

Pic. 2 COWON D2 MP3 player, which I used.

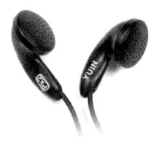

Pic. 3 YUIN PK2 headphones - APPROPRIATE
Not inserted deep in ear. I used this model.

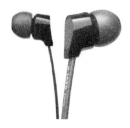

Pic. 4 JAYS earphones called "earplugs" – inserted deep in ear. DO NOT USE. As they are plugged in ears, they reduce sounds from the environment.

I don't recommend using mobile phones, Bluetooth, on-ear, or earplugs headphones, as using mobile phones with Bluetooth headphones for TRT therapy, because:
- The phone's limited range of volume, which typically only have 15 levels of volume instead of the usual 50 or 100.
- Additionally, it is recommended to use wired headphones as Bluetooth technology emits radiation. Consistent exposure to this for 8 hours a day, especially near the brain, may have effects on your health.
- If you choose to use an mp3 player, you can download Pink Noise for free from my web. This is Pink noise which many others used during recovery. Pink noise and white noise are both effective for tinnitus retraining therapy, regardless of whether or not you experience hyperacusis.

Second option - TRT Noise Generator - Audiofon, Siemens, or Phonak. The Siemens model costs around 420 USD and the Audiofon around 200 USD, Phonak around 300 USD (Phonak are good for people with hearing loss). The price is for one piece. They look a bit like hearing aids.

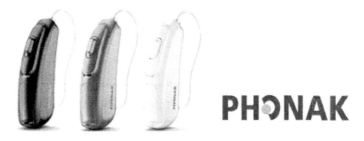

Pic. 1 Phonak Pink & White Noise Generators

"Opposing Opinion" from Michaela N.:

Because I have a personal experience with Siemens noise generators mentioned by Peter, Besides the disadvantages, I found them to be more user friendly, but it is a purely subjective view. The entry investment is not small, but if the sufferer avoids spending on ineffective methods of treatment or preparations, those headphones are not a waste of money. For example, I do not mind the wearing of the hearing aid; on the contrary, it was rather complicated use my MP3, probably also because I was not used to listening to music on one. The big advantage of this system is the remote control, where it is possible to adjust the volume according to the ascending line 0-12 for each ear, and to monitor the improvement. I want to say that I like sound generators more, even though I admire his idea with mp3 player. But for those who do not have the mp3 player and do not mind that they will have a noise generator behind the ear (the end cap in the ear is not visible), they do not have to worry about those hearing aids.

HOW TO GET REQUIRED TIME

You need to hear it eight hours per day. And it takes an average 1,5 years to heal completely. However, I felt good results after two weeks of strict adherence. How to listen to noise 8 hours a day?

I got up in the morning, I just took my MP3 player and set the volume. I listened until I got to work – while eating, brushing my teeth, dressing, and traveling, etc. This alone was about 2 hours each morning. Because I was working in a management position, I couldn't listen to the headphones at work. But when I left work, I started to listen the noise again and listened from 5:00 pm to 11:00 pm until I went to sleep. So altogether, this was 8 hours, as required. Nowadays, it's great that the earphones are small, and many people listen to an MP3, so you will not feel abnormal and no one will be looking at you strangely.

You set the intensity of the noise every morning when you are in a quiet place, and on that day, you will NEVER change it. It does not matter that you will not hear this noise in the subway or in the pub. The brain will perceive it even though the noise of the pub or subway is stronger

DAILY TINNITUS MEASUREMENT

"Turn your SHOULDs into MUSTs."

Tony Robbins

Knowing that the problem is not in your ear (you have undergone neurological and ORL examinations) and you are completely "healthy," you need to repair the unconscious filters in your brain. TRT therapy uses pink or white noise because these sounds can distract the brain from tinnitus.

Regularly listening to pink noise (the differences are explained earlier in the hyperacusis chapter), the brain completely stops perceiving tinnitus. This means tinnitus will completely disappear from your life, and after the treatment time you will not need to listen to anything else and you can return to the state you were in before you had tinnitus.

It is very important to observe some rules when listening to pink noise. The first and most important thing is that the noise level must be lower than the volume of the tinnitus. The second most important thing is that the brain perceives the noise for an enough time per day. In the past, similar sounds were to be used to mask tinnitus, but the noise was higher than tinnitus. This method provided relief for the patient, but their tinnitus was not cured. Therefore, I repeat once again, the volume of tinnitus must be higher than the volume of noise. In other words, when listening to noise, you must clearly hear tinnitus as well. When you get up in the morning, take the MP3 player. Sit on the bed and set the volume. In silence, see if you can also hear your tinnitus. If not, reduce the volume of the noise until you can clearly hear it. Setup pink or white noise as low as audible. At the same time, you need to hear tinnitus clearly. Do not adjust the intensity during the day. If the tinnitus in each ear is heard with a different intensity on the MP3 player, adjust the volume for each ear by the "balance" function (ask the store if the player has the function). If your tinnitus is different in each ear, make sure that the player allows it before purchasing. Some Cowon and Fiio players have this feature.

If your tinnitus is lower one day, you will be able to hear pink noise on lower volume level.

If your tinnitus will be higher other day, you will need to increase volume of pink noise to hear pink noise.

This is an indirect, objective and quite precise way to measure volume of your tinnitus every day.

Setup volume of pink noise every day in the morning to LOWEST audible volume. Your tinnitus MUST be always much louder. Setup volume 15 minutes after you wake up (your brain is fully wakened up) in a quiet room. Volume will vary from day to day and this will help you to find things, situations and people, which makes your tinnitus louder and which makes it lower.

During the day, you may notice that you are not able to hear pink noise, because of the surrounding noise (cars, colleagues, restaurant). It is ok and do not increase the volume of the pink noise. Your brain is perceiving it.

Example of how-to setup the volume of PINK NOISE:
The starting volume of PINK NOISE is for example 10.
- Pink noise volume 10. You hear tinnitus and pink noise.
  Action: Decrease the volume of pink noise to 9.
- Pink noise volume 9. You hear tinnitus and pink noise.
  Action: Decrease the volume of pink noise to 8.
- Pink noise volume 8. You hear tinnitus and pink noise.
  Action: Decrease the volume of pink noise to 7.
- Pink noise volume 7. You hear tinnitus only. You don't hear pink noise at tall.
  Action: Increase the volume of pink noise to 8.
- Now you had setup pink noise on lowest audible volume

level.

Action 1) Don't change volume all day and listen to the pink noise 8 hours.

Action 2) Write the lowest audible volume of pink noise in your tinnitus diary. You will see how your tinnitus is changing and decreasing.

Again: by setting the volume of pink noise at the LOWEST AUDIBLE volume every morning, I also measured the volume of my tinnitus on that day.

When my tinnitus was strong that morning, I had to raise the volume of pink noise in the morning to make the pink noise audible at all.

When my tinnitus was quieter another day, I could also decrease the volume of pink noise.

This way, I measured my tinnitus volume every day.

TINNITUS DIARY

TINNITUS DIARY AND HOW TO FIND WHAT IS MAKING YOUR TINNITUS WORSE AND WHAT MAKES IT BETTER

"Insanity is doing the same thing over and over and expecting different results."

Albert Einstein

Tinnitus diary is available here for free download on my web: www.icuredmytinnitus.com

Every morning I wrote down the volume of my tinnitus in my tinnitus diary. In the morning, I sat on the bed (15 minutes after I woke up) I adjusted the volume of noise (as instructed at the end of the previous chapter) and I knew exactly if tinnitus was stronger or weaker that the day before. When I had to increase volume of pink noise to be able to hear pink noise at all, I knew that tinnitus was also stronger, that day.

When I heard pink noise on lower volume, I knew that tinnitus is weaker at that day. This is how I was able to measure the volume of my tinnitus every day.

Important notice again - tinnitus MUST be always much louder, than pink noise. Pink noise needs to be listened on lowest possible volume and this will vary every day.

I also saw the tendency of descending as weeks passed by. In addition to the volume, I also recorded what I drank and ate the day before. After one month, I exactly knew what drinks and foods made my tinnitus stronger and I excluded them from my life. Later I also wrote in my diary the situations I experienced and the people I met, the day before. Sit on your bed, setup the volume of pink/white noise to lowest audible volume. Write down the volume and what you ate and drank the day before. After one month, write down also what you did and who you met the day before. Every two weeks, mark days with high tinnitus volume and find common signs of those days (i.e., FRIED food, alcohol, food FLAVORS and ingredients, canned food, non-washed vegetables and fruits, sports, work, people). Also find out what makes your tinnitus lower. In my case it was sauna, reading, lens and beans. Using the diary, I received: Accurate daily measurement of the volume of my tinnitus, I have seen how the volume of tinnitus decreases over time, the descending measured tendency has calmed me much, I have clearly seen that I my tinnitus volume is decreasing, and I am going to heal I exactly knew what increases and what decreases my tinnitus: What food, What drinks, Which situations, Which people.

Because I knew exactly what made it worse and what helped me, I knew what food and drink I needed to omit, and on the contrary, what food and drink I should eat and drink more. As I did this, my tinnitus volume quickly dropped and did not return to high volumes. Other things which became clear were situations and people, which made my tinnitus worse. For example, it was roller skating, meeting my parents, stress at work, and so on. For roller skating I consulted this whit physiotherapist, who helped me with body posture and then it was ok. For meeting parents, stress at work, fear (psychological consequences), I consulted with my psychologist and opened my trauma from childhood which needs to be healed. I did have need to check my tinnitus several times during the day, because I knew exactly if my tinnitus was weaker or stronger as day before.

The diary of the tinnitus shortened my treatment from a year and a half to nine months. When it is done honestly and all things which are found are resolved, most of the people who are consulting me are tinnitus free within a few months. So, write the diary regularly. It will take you five minutes a day and the benefits are great. Also find the courage to solve the situations that will show up. For example, on beginning I was very ashamed to contact psychologist, but at the end it helped me so much, not only cure the tinnitus, but also to live a much healthier life.

1. I have seen how the volume of tinnitus decreases over time, the descending measured tendency has calmed me much, I have clearly seen that my tinnitus volume is decreasing, and I am going to heal.

2. I exactly knew what increases and what decreases my tinnitus:
   a. What food,
   b. What drinks,
   c. Which situations,
   d. Which people.

As I knew exactly what made my tinnitus worse and what helped me, I knew what food and drink I needed to omit, and on the contrary, what food and drink I should eat and drink more. As I did this, my tinnitus volume quickly dropped and did not return to high volumes. Other things which became clear were situations and people, which made my tinnitus worse. For example, it was roller skating, meeting my parents, stress at work, and so on. For roller skating I consulted this with my physiotherapist, who helped me with body posture and then roller skating was ok. As for meeting parents, stress at work, fear (psychological consequences), I consulted with psychologist and together, we opened my trauma from childhood which needed to be healed.

3. I didn't have need to check my tinnitus several times during the day, because I knew exactly if my tinnitus was weaker or stronger as compared to the day before. This helped me to pay much less attention to my tinnitus.

The diary of the tinnitus shortened my treatment from a year and a half to nine months. When it is done honestly and all things which are found are resolved, most of the people who are consulting me are tinnitus free within a few months. So, fill in your diary every day. It will take you five minutes a day and the benefits are great. Also, find the courage to solve those personal situations that will show up.

For example, in the beginning I was very ashamed to contact psychologists, but in the end, it helped me so much, not only was I able to cure the tinnitus, but also to have a much better life.

During the first month, every morning I wrote down in my diary:
- The lowest audible volume of pink noise and,
- what I ate and drank during this first month.

After two weeks in the first month, and then every two weeks, I marked with a red highlighter the days when I had tinnitus strong (for example, values 17, 15, 14, 18) and identified those common things for these different days at the different values. This way I determined the meals and drinks that strengthened my tinnitus. Then I marked with a green highlighter the days when my tinnitus was weak (for example, values 12, 10, 9, 11) and looked for common things for these days. This way, I found food and drink that improved my condition, made my tinnitus weaker.

I stopped eating and drinking things that strengthened my tinnitus and I started eating and drinking more things which weakened my tinnitus (in the diet chapter I described it in detail which of those things they were).

The second month, after I adjusted my diet, I continued the same way, and in addition to writing down my meals and drinks, I started writing down my daily activities and the people which I met the day before. By doing so, I have been able to find out which activities and people were strengthening my tinnitus, and which were reducing my tinnitus. I readdressed those findings with the psychologist and the physiotherapist until I have become completely cured (in the chapter psychology, I write about this in detail).

It helped me a lot to see how my tinnitus volume went down over time

STEP FOUR

STRESS, EMOTIONAL RELIEF AND HOW TO GET PROPER SLEEP DURING RECOVERY.

PSYCHOLOGY AND STRESS RELIEF

"Our only obligation is to always be true to ourselves and to allow."

Anita Moorjani

Find someone you trust and with whom you can share your troubles. I personally recommend the following books: *"Drama of the gifted child"* by Alice Miller; *"In an unspoken voice"* by Dr. Peter Levine. There was a need to find the psychosomatic cause of my tinnitus. I myself have made great changes in my life and I would say that my successful cure was in large part a result of the combination of TRT therapy and psychosomatic help. I describe the changes in my life at the end of the book.

From a psychosomatic point of view, it is necessary to focus on finding the psychological cause of your tinnitus, such as anxiety. The aim is to understand what we do "wrong" or what we do not do and what we should do - a malfunctioning model of our behavior. This malfunction causes much stress, and we already know this increases the volume of one's tinnitus. Only when we really understand what the problem is, can we understand why tinnitus is perceived (every person in the world has it, but most do not even know it). When you "put together" your life, you will stop hearing tinnitus, as people "without tinnitus".

Common Psychosomatic Causes:
- Closing out of the sounds from the outside (lots of information, often negative or unpleasant – e.g., constant remorse from a partner).
- Anxiety - focusing on inner sounds, frequent observations (for example, based on an unpleasant experience when our problems have long been distorted or worsened).
- Reluctance to listen to criticism (one does not want to hear what he or she cannot defend or respond to - such as criticism from the boss).

- Inability to hear an inner voice (for example, we know that the work does not suit us, but we do not do anything about it).
- Another thing that is common during consultations is a certain hardness and the inability to cry. This was true in my situation. I did not cry for 18 years, because crying was not "manly." So, if you cry, you have a great chance of getting rid of tinnitus simply by allowing yourself to cry. When crying, you will also clean your cavities and relax pressure in them, because after the crying, everybody will need to blow their nose. I personally did not cry for 18 years before tinnitus, and when I learned to cry again, it helped me a lot. The ears, neck and nose are closely connected and interacting with each other.
- The last thing is rage. I do not know if you can generalize it, but when I solved my rage it helped me a lot. When I was unable to resist criticism, I was inwardly upset and noticed that in my sleep I gritted my teeth. Gritting of the teeth is a clear manifestation of unsolved rage. When your jaws are clenched, you will increase your tinnitus. Try it and you will see that when jaws are clenched, tinnitus is louder. When I solved my inner rage, and released it, my jaws relaxed, and my tinnitus dropped again.

Understanding and solving psychological consequences was an essential part of my cure. As you see, it is no miracle, but normal biological patterns. My cure had several components that had to be followed until I was completely cured. I believe you will also find your way to your complete cure. Try to take tinnitus as an indication that something is wrong in your life and you just need to resolve it to be healthy. To understand your own story and the psychological consequences that tinnitus can relate to, I recommend reading these books, which helped me a lot:

Dr. Alice Miller (Swiss psychologist)
Book - Drama of a gifted child

Dr. Peter A. Levine (American Scientist and Psychologist)
Book – In an unspoken voice

Dr. Bessel van der Kolk MD
Book - The Body Keeps the Score

SLEEPING RECOMMENDATIONS

The next thing is adequate sleep. Go to bed so you sleep for at least 8 hours. If you cannot sleep, read a nice book before sleep, as it will help to calm you down and help you fall sleep. Before going to bed, take an hour for walking, listening to calming music, reading a nice book. Before bedtime, do not eat anything heavy: ideally, you should eat a big lunch and a smaller dinner. When you wake up on the weekend, read in bed and maybe you will go back to sleep again. When you get home tired, do not have coffee or black/green tea, but take a nap for at least half an hour.

Other recommendations for better sleep:
- **Avoid silence** and use sound enrichment to be surrounded by pleasant sounds while you sleep. It could be nature sounds which come thought window, refrigerator, aquarium or any other sounds.
  - I listened to aquarium and fridge which were close to my sleeping room.
  - Our windows were opened for micro-ventilation always, so I could hear noise from the street.
- When using a computer before sleep, **I used f.lux program** (free), or night shift on Mac, or phone.
- It also worked for me in the evening by **flushing my ears with clean water.**
- Every day I used to **read a book before sleep.**
- When I woke up and could not sleep again.
  - I **wrote every thought and idea to my diary**, which I always kept next to my bed.
  - I start to read my book again.
- Understand that you can cure your tinnitus.
- After every **emotional release** I used to get a good sleep.
- I didn't exercise, work, watch or read any *"dramas"* two hours before sleep.

- I you really struggling with sleep, please find sleeping specialist and read great book – Why we sleep, by Matthew Walker. Here are his 12 key tips:

1. Stick to a sleep schedule
We should aim to go to bed and wake up at the same time each day. People generally have a hard time adjusting to changes in sleep patterns. Unfortunately sleeping late on weekends doesn't make up for poor sleep during the week. If necessary, set an alarm for bedtime. Matthew emphasises this is the #1 priority from the list; stick to a regular sleep schedule.

2. Don't exercise too late in the day
Exercise is great, and we should try to exercise at least 30 minutes on most days. But try to time it no later than 2-3 hours before bed.

3. Avoid caffeine & nicotine
Colas, coffee, teas (that aren't herbal), and chocolate contain caffeine, which is a stimulant. Even consuming these in the afternoon can have an effect on your sleep. Nicotine is also a mild stimulant, and smokers will often wake up earlier than they would otherwise, due to nicotine withdrawal.

4. Avoid alcoholic drinks before bed
The presence of alcohol in the body can reduce your REM sleep, keeping you in the lighter stages of sleep.

5. Avoid large meals and beverages late at night
A lights snack before bed is okay, but a heavy meal can cause digestive issues, which interferes with sleep. Drinking too many fluids can cause frequent awakenings to urinate.

6. Avoid medicines that delay or disrupt your sleep (where possible)
Some commonly prescribed medications, even for tinnitus, as well as some over the counter and herbal medicines can disrupt sleep patterns. If you have trouble sleeping, it may be worth speaking to your doctor to see if any of the drugs you're taking

may be contributing to this. It may be possible to take them earlier in the day.

7. Don't nap after 3pm
Naps are great, but taking them too late in the day can make it hard to fall asleep at night.

8. Make sure to leave time to relax before bed
It's important to have time before bed to unwind. Try to schedule your days so that there is time to relax before bed.

9. Take a hot bath before bed
The drop in body temperature after a bath may help you to feel sleepy, and the bath can help you to slow down and relax before bed. This is what helped me most.

10. Have a dark, cool (in temperature), gadget free bedroom
We sleep better at night if the temperature in the room is kept on the cool side. Gadgets such as mobile phones and computers can be a distraction. Additionally the light they emit, especially the blue light, suppresses the secretion of melatonin. Melatonin being a hormone that regulates sleep/wake cycles – with it increasing in the evening to induce sleep. There are things we can do to reduce the blue light at night, including:

- Already mentioned, using blue light filters on our phones & tablets and PC or MAC. It is called Night Shift, Twilight, f.lux, Night Light.
- Using blue light filters on our home lighting system.
- A comfortable mattress and pillow can set you up for a good sleep. Those with insomnia will often watch the clock, turn it away from view so you don't have to worry about the time while trying to sleep. Use these tips to optimise your sleeping space.

11. Get the right sunlight exposure
Sun exposure during the day helps us to regulate sleeping patterns. Try to get outside in the natural sunlight for at least 30 minutes per day.

12. Don't stay in bed if you (really) can't sleep
If you find yourself still in bed for more than 20 minutes, or you're starting to get anxious in bed, get up and do something else until you feel sleepy. Anxiety whilst trying to sleep can make it harder to fall asleep.

STEP FIVE

FIX YOU BODY POSTURE, SPINE AND JAWS WITH PHYSIOTHERAPIST AND MOVEMENT.

SPINE AND JAWS

After I had confirmation that I don't have any physiological reason, I started with therapy. During the therapy I realised that some positions of my jaws and body increase my tinnitus. Also, I found out that roller-skating and swimming increase it (I described this in chapter *Tinnitus diary*). I found a great physiotherapist and we started to work on body postures and unblocking my cervical spine and jaws. After some time, roller-skating and swimming didn't increase my tinnitus anymore. Also, I found out that when I was cold, my tinnitus increased. I started to clean my sinusitis in cooperation with an ENT specialist. It was done by salt water (organic salt and boiled/cold water). When I cleaned my nose every day, I stopped to get cold and my tinnitus was little bit weaker.

EXERCISE AND BODY

Movement. Regular, no overload. So, fitness, bicycle, skating, dancing, skiing, tennis. Whatever you like. I would avoid noisy motorsports and football matches.

Here are some general physiotherapy recommendations:

- Walking instead of using the elevator, walking after work.
- Swimming, mainly on your back.
- Dance.
- Make breaks while working on your computer, every hour for 10 minutes.
- Massage your upper back.
- Set the right seating position for your computer.
- As mentioned about check your spine and jaws with a good physiotherapist.

If you cannot move because you struggle with pain I highly recommend books by Pete Egosque.

STEP SIX

MANY MEALS MAY MAKE YOUR TINNITUS LOUDER, WHILE OTHERS MAY HELP TO REDUCE ITS INTENSITY.

DIET CHANGE

"No matter where we live on the planet or how difficult our situation seems to be, we have the ability to overcome and transcend our circumstances."

Louise Hay

DIET RECOMMENDATION

I will not persuade you to make a radical change to your diet, but try to eat more salads, fruits and vegetables. If you can, omit fast food, everything fried, cola, coffee and cigarettes. Instead of eating sweets, eat fruit. Drink alcohol only on special occasions. When you are cured, you will not have to drink sorrow, and it be worth it.

Drinks
- Drink hot water and herbal teas (before going to sleep, for example, a calming tea)
- Filter tap water (using a Brita filter or a similar brand).
- Skip alcohol, sweet drinks, non-alcoholic beer and juices in a box.

Foods
- Eat lots of vegetables - fresh and frozen.
- Eat fruit for dessert (wash every food properly and if possible, eat organic fruits and vegetables only).
- Eat raw nuts (not fried, etc.).
- Eat fish and white meat (turkey, duck, chicken) a few times a week.
- Skip fried, sweet, pork, beef, sausages, avocados, cheeses, chocolate, raisins and dates.
- Limit bread, salt, and dairy.

These dietary restrictions are only required during therapy: after your therapy is completed, it is possible to start to eat some of the previously restricted items again.

The aim is to eliminate foods that irritate the nervous system, such as sugar, heavy metals, alcohol, caffeine, or those containing tyramine.

I have noticed that tinnitus is very often perceived as "stronger" because of these foods. You can also trace what foods irritate your nervous system, meaning if the tinnitus volume is higher, the day after that particular food was eaten, you can now identify what foods and/or drink to stop eating. You now should omit these foods and drinks. Sometimes one simple food is enough to irritate you, therefore, increasing the perception of tinnitus.

Here are the top 10 foods you should always try to avoid during recovery:
- Margarine – Your brain requires fats to make new brain cells. Fats aren't inherently bad. In fact, they are essential, but the quality of those fats can alter the ease of cell-to-cell communication within your brain. In contrast, fats like Omega 3s improve functioning. Extra virgin olive oil is an excellent alternative that has been shown to improve brain health.
- Table Salt – Swap out your table salt for some Pink Himalayan sea salt. Table salt is bleached and heavily processed. Pink Himalayan sea salts will give you more of what your body needs.
- Fruit Juice/Soda – These sugar-laden drinks spike your sugar levels.
- Microwaved Foods – Avoid the radiation of microwaves. Don't stand near them if they're on. I gave away my microwave.
- Farm-raised Fish Like Salmon. The best option is to try Alaskan wild-caught Salmon.
- Factory Farmed Meats – These meats are higher in chemicals. Find a source you can visit such as a local farm, not a factory, and talk directly to the farmer. Local farms are more likely to have healthier chickens and eggs, too.
- Artificial Sweeteners – Sugar-free does not mean it's healthier. Stick with the sugar but limit the amount you eat. Remember the mantra, "Everything in moderation." Or try locally sourced raw honey that offers a little added protection specific to your area.
- Processed Foods Containing Colourings & Dyes – These dyes dramatically affect your brain and tinnitus.
- Processed Meat is LOADED with preservatives. This can affect

your brain and increase tinnitus.

"The Dirty Dozen" – These 12 foods have the highest concentration of chemicals: Strawberries, Spinach, Nectarines, Apples, Peaches, Pears, Cherries, Grapes, Celery, Tomatoes, Sweet Bell Peppers, and Potatoes. This beautiful variety of foods is polluted with chemicals. Only buy these foods if they are organic. When choosing between organic foods and non-organic, these are the scariest.

Choose the "Clean 15" instead: Sweet Corn, Avocado, Pineapples, Cabbage, Onions, Frozen Sweet Peas, Papayas, Asparagus, Mangos, Eggplant, Honeydew, Kiwi, Cantaloupe, Cauliflower, and Grapefruit.

Plus I highly recommend avoiding wheat (gluten), sugar (including sweeteners), and dairy (specially cow).

TIP: Clean properly every vegetable and fruit before eating.

In my case, I had to avoid also bananas, avocados, apples, alcohol (except cider), chocolate, and sweets, because I found that, these foods are increasing my tinnitus. You could have different ones. I found it during daily tinnitus measurement and with the help of a tinnitus diary.

Find yours with Tinnitus Diary. You can download Tinnitus Diary for free from my web: www.icuredmytinnitus.com

HYPERACUSIS

For those who have tinnitus, because of an acoustic trauma (loud noise), any sound will cause them pain. Hyperacusis is a very high sensitivity to sounds. In my case, when I was in a quiet room and someone was reading a newspaper there and reversing the pages, the sound was so intense to me, that I could not stand it. In restaurants, in the subway, and so on, all the sounds were unbearable to me, and it hurt terribly. If you have a similar problem, this chapter is for you.

If you also suffer from hyperacusis, the good news is that you will treat the hyperacusis the same way as tinnitus. The only difference is that instead of white noise you will be listening to pink noise. Pink noise has cropped high frequencies, making it much softer for listening.

The following two pictures graphically illustrate the difference between white and pink noise.

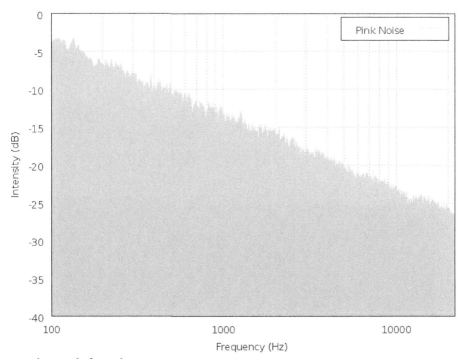

Pic. 5 Pink noise

In the picture with pink noise, you can see that the intensity gradually decreases with frequency. High frequencies (such as train whistles, opera singers, or applause) are very uncomfortable for people with hyperacusis and therefore pink noise is used in TRT therapy for hyperacusis. Pink noise cures both tinnitus and hyperacusis at the same time. Because I suffered from hyperacusis, I used pink noise during my therapy.

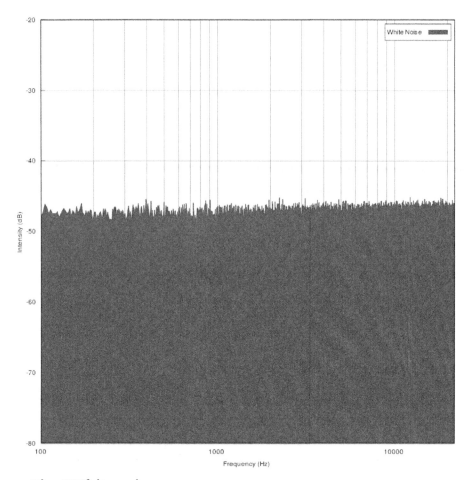

Pic. 6 White noise

For white noise, you can see that all frequencies have the same volume. I tried white noise, but I was uncomfortable to listen, so I did not use it anymore.

I recommend using pink noise because:
- It has same healing effect as white noise, ever if you have not hyperacusis
- You can download pink noise from my web for free and this pink noise is tested.

In addition to listening to pink noise instead of white noise, there are a few more rules that needs to be followed temporarily:

- Avoid loud spaces such as theatres, cinemas, restaurants, demonstrations, etc.
- In cases where you cannot avoid it, wear earplugs in noisy areas for 1.5 months. When you leave the noisy environment, for example, get off the subway, put earplugs off and start to listen to pink noise.
- 2nd month cut the earplugs in half (lengthwise, not width) and in noisy environments, wear them as before. It could be unpleasant at first, but it's like when you remove a plaster after a fracture, and you must start rehabilitation. You will still avoid rock concerts, F1 races, live football and hockey games at stadiums, celebrations with fireworks, cinemas, theatres and so on.
- 3rd month, you can stop using the earplugs. Give yourself two more months and do not expose your ears to a concert, and so on.
- At the end of your therapy, have earplugs always in your pockets and always use them in theatres, concerts, motor races, hockey, on New Year's Eve, etc. You do not need it just because you had tinnitus and hyperacusis, but because you love yourself and don't want to damage your ears again. You can also recommend them to every friend. All the big events are terribly overcrowded and the sound so high that it can destroy one's hearing.

FREQUENTLY ASKED QUESTIONS

Q: COULD YOU PLEASE RECOMMEND ME A DEVICE FOR PINK/WHITE NOISE LISTENING?

You can find the best combination tested on my web.

Q: HOW SHOULD I DO TRT THERAPY CORRECTLY?
- This is a detailed description with examples, of how to set up the volume of TRT therapy: The default volume setting is for example 10 (the default volume will vary):
- You hear tinnitus and you also hear pink/white noise = you decrease the volume of pink/white noise to volume 9.
- You hear tinnitus and you also hear pink/white noise – you decrease the volume of pink/white noise to volume 8.
- You hear tinnitus and you also hear pink/white noise – you decrease the volume of pink/white noise to volume 7.
- You hear tinnitus and youI also hear pink/white noise – you decrease the volume of pink/white noise to volume 6.
- You hear tinnitus and you cannot hear pink/white noise – you increase the volume of pink/white noise to volume 7.
- Then I do not change the volume all day and you listen to it 8 hours.
- You write the volume value in the tinnitus diary, so you see the progres.

Q: SHOULD THE TINNITUS SOUND BE LOUDER THAN PINK/WHITE NOISE?
Yes, tinnitus sound must be always louder than pink/white noise.

Q: IS LISTENING TO THE WHITE/PINK NOISE, THE MORE THE BETTER? DOES IT MAKE SENSE TO LISTEN TO IT FOR MORE THAN 8 HOURS A DAY?
8 hours a day is ideal. Neither more nor less.

Q: IS IT NECESSARY TO LISTEN TO WHITE/PINK NOISE THROUGH THE HEADPHONES OR IS IT POSSIBLE TO LISTEN TO IT THROUGH THE SPEAKERS?
You have to listen through headphones.

Q: IS IT POSSIBLE TO LISTEN DURING THE NIGHT WHILE YOU ARE ASLEEP?
You need to listen during the day.

Q: IS IT NECESSARY TO CHOOSE ONE SOUND AND LISTEN TO IT CONSISTENTLY OR CAN IT BE CHANGED?
I recommend one, ideally good white or pink noise. It is important that noise has very good quality.

Q: I'M NOT SURE HOW TO SET THE VOLUME BECAUSE I HAVE THE TINNITUS IN THE LEFT EAR-NOT IN THE RIGHT AND YES IT DOES CALM ME DOWN.
If you have tinnitus in only one ear, you can use just one headphone or adjust the balance settings on your player to use one side only. Using both headphones is also an option, but keep in mind that the volume of the pink noise should be set to the lowest possible level. Tinnitus should always be much louder than the background noise. You can download pink noise for free from this website, which I personally used and many others have had success with.

Q: HOW TINNITUS DIARY HELPED YOU?
Every morning, I recorded the volume of my tinnitus in my tinnitus diary using sound therapy to measure it. I sat on my bed and adjusted the volume of noise to determine whether the tinnitus was stronger or weaker than the previous day. Over time, I noticed a downward trend in the volume of my tinnitus.

Additionally, I recorded what I ate and drank the day before to identify any foods or drinks that made my tinnitus worse. By eliminating these items from my diet, I was able to reduce the severity of my tinnitus. I also started writing down the situations and people I encountered each day to further identify any triggers that worsened my tinnitus. This diary was a helpful tool in managing my tinnitus. Using the tinnitus diary given to me:
Accurate daily measurement of the volume of my tinnitus,
I have seen how the volume of tinnitus decreases over time, and the descending measured tendency has calmed me much, I have clearly seen that my tinnitus volume is decreasing and I am going to heal.

I exactly knew what increases and what decreases my tinnitus:
- What food,
- What drinks,
- Which situations,
- Which people.

I did not need to check my tinnitus several times during the day because I knew exactly if my tinnitus was weaker or stronger than the day before.

By keeping a tinnitus diary, I was able to identify triggers that worsened my tinnitus and make lifestyle changes accordingly. I knew which foods and drinks to avoid and which to consume more of, and I also discovered that certain situations and people made my tinnitus worse. For example, roller skating caused my tinnitus to worsen, but consulting with a physiotherapist helped me correct my body posture and alleviate the issue. I also sought help from a psychologist to address psychological triggers, such as stress at work and trauma from childhood.

Checking my tinnitus volume every day helped me track its progress and adjust my therapy accordingly. By consistently using the diary, I was able to shorten my treatment from a year and a half to just nine months. For example, thanx to Tinnitu Diary I discovered that roller skating caused my tinnitus to worsen, but consulting with a physiotherapist helped me correct my body posture and alleviate the issue. I also sought help from a psychologist to address psychological triggers, such as stress at work and trauma from childhood. I encourage others to keep a tinnitus diary as well, as it only takes a few minutes a day and can lead to significant benefits. While I may not have been meticulous about recording every detail of my daily life, I made sure to include the most important information, such as any special meals, junk food, alcohol, and sweets that I consumed.

Q: DO I HAVE TO LISTEN TO PINK OR WHITE NOISE EVERY DAY FOR 8 HOURS? WHAT IF, FOR EXAMPLE, ONE DAY I WILL LISTEN 5 HOURS, ANOTHER 4 HOURS, AND THE NEXT 10 HOURS? (OVER THE WEEKEND, I HAVE MORE TIME TO LISTEN TO IT)
You can listen less then 8 hours, but do not listen more 8 hours. In time try to manage your day, so you can listen approximately 8 hours a day.

Q: CAN I SKIP A DAY, OR TWO? (FOR EXAMPLE, FOR TWO DAYS ON A RAFT). WHAT WILL HAPPEN IF I MISS ONE DAY?
Yes you can. For example, skipping one day has no effect on therapy. Important is what you do regularly, not occasionally.

Q: WHAT HEADPHONES DO I NEED TO USE?
Please refer to my web where are regular updated available sound therapy devices.

Q: CAN I LISTEN TO A PINK NOISE EVEN WHEN I HAVE NO HYPERACUSIS?
Yes, you can. It is equally effective as White Noise. You can download Pink Noise for free from my web.

CAN I HEAR PINK NOISE ON THE SPEAKER OVERNIGHT - SOMEWHERE NEAR MY HEAD? WILL IT BE A PARTIAL REPLACEMENT FOR TINNITUS SOUND THERAPY?
No. At night for better sleep, use sound enrichment.

Q: WHAT IS MORE IMPORTANT? DIET OR SOUND THERAPY?

Both, and in my case, stress relief was a big part of the complete tinnitus relief.

Q: USING YOUR TECHNIQUE IN THE BOOK, I ARRIVED AT A VOLUME SETTING OF 9 WHERE I COULD HEAR NO PINK NOISE, BUT TINNITUS. HOWEVER, THE PINK NOISE AT 10 IS JUST DETECTABLE, AND I MEAN JUST. AM I RIGHT IN UNDERSTANDING THAT I SHOULD STAY ON 10 RATHER THAN UPPING IT ONE TO 11?

A: Yes, at this case please stay at volume level 10.

HI PETER I BOUGHT YOUR BOOK AND IT IS VERY HELPFUL. I WAS WONDERING IF I COULD PLAY PINK NOISE THROUGH A BOSE SPEAKER - IE AT NIGHT AND DURING THE DAY - INSTEAD OF LISTENING TO IT WITH AN MP3 PLAYER AND HEADPHONES. I FIND PINK NOISE CALMS ME DOWN A LOT. THANK YOU FOR ALL YOUR HELP.

It is recommended to use an MP3 player for TRT therapy. Pink noise has two benefits: it can help calm you down, and when used with an MP3 player and headphones, it can also help break fixation on tinnitus. In my case, my tinnitus changed over time with the use of pink noise and as it helped calm me down, I was eventually cured and the volume decreased to a non-audible level. Using an MP3 player can also help you keep track of your tinnitus diary and support your recovery. It's important to only listen to pink noise during the day, as your brain needs to rest at night. For sound enrichment, you can use pink noise through your speakers.

Q: I DON'T HAVE AN OBJECTIVE CAUSE FOR TINNITUS BUT I HAD DONE A TEST LIKE YOU KNOW HEARING TEST WITH AN AUDIOLOGIST AND IT SHOWED SOME HAIR CELLS NOT RESPONDING ON HIGH FREQUENCIES AND I HAVE VERY LIGHT HEARING LOSS, SO IS THIS AN OBJECTIVE REASON OR THIS IS NO PROBLEM FOR YOUR THERAPY?

Partial loss of hearing is not a problem for therapy. You just need to adjust the volume for each ear separately.

Q: DID YOU HAVE ANY SETBACKS? AS YOU KNOW TINNITUS STARTED TO LOWER VOLUME AND AFTER A COUPLE OF DAYS, IT STARTED TO BUZZ MORE. FOR EXAMPLE, I CUT DOWN ON SUGAR SALT AND I HAVE NO EFFECT ON LOWERING T.

I have encountered setbacks. However, it is not uncommon, and as a precautionary measure, I document all details in my tinnitus diary. By referring to my tinnitus diary, I could make necessary changes in my lifestyle to avoid further setbacks. Nevertheless, it is imperative to use a device to measure tinnitus, without the aid of a measuring device, any changes may not be noticeable.

Q: DID YOU HAVE ANY HEARING LOSS?

Yes, I had, caused by acoustic trauma. Most of my hearing was recovered.

Q: BEFORE DOING SOUND THERAPY DO I NEED TO SEE A SPECIALIST TO TELL ME WHAT DB MY TINNITUS IS ITS FREQUENCY/S AND WHICH SIDE IT IS ON, LEFT OR RIGHT, AND AT WHAT VOLUME, ETC.?

A: No, you just need to see a specialist to exclude objective reason.

Q: CAN I USE PINK NOISE OR IS WHITE NOISE BETTER? DOES IT MATTER?

Pink noise and White noise are equally effective. So please use Pink noise from my site, which was used by me and many others with good results.

Q: DURING THE DAY I CAN DISTRACT MYSELF FROM THE NOISE IF I AM BUSY AND THERE ARE SOUNDS FROM THE ENVIRONMENT I.E CRICKETS/WIND ETC. ONLY WHEN I SIT IN A QUIET/RELATIVELY QUIET ROOM IT CAN BECOME LOUD AND INTRUSIVE, DO I STILL NEED SOUND THERAPY?

Ideally, you should not hear tinnitus in a quiet environment as well. So yes.

Q: WHAT DO YOU THINK ABOUT SOUND NOTCH THERAPY?

I do not have any experience with notch therapy.

Q: HI PETER, I'VE BEEN READING YOUR BOOK, AND GOING THROUGH YOUR WEBSITE AND FACEBOOK PAGE. I HAD A FEW QUESTIONS AS I'M GOING THROUGH IT. IN YOUR BOOK, FOR TRT YOU MENTION LISTENING TO PINK NOISE IF YOU HAVE TINNITUS AND HYPERACUSIS, AND YOU SAY YOU SHOULD LISTEN TO WHITE NOISE IF YOU ONLY HAVE TINNITUS. HOWEVER, ON YOUR WEBSITE, IT SAYS TO LISTEN TO PINK NOISE FOR TINNITUS. SO IF YOU ONLY HAVE TINNITUS, WHICH TYPE OF NOISE SHOULD YOU USE? WHITE OR PINK?

Hello pink and white noise are equally effective even if you don't have hyperacusis. Pink noise on my site is tested hence I recommend that for you.

Q: IF MY TINNITUS IS AT A DIFFERENT LEVEL IN EACH EAR, IS IT OKAY IF THE WHITE/PINK NOISE IS AT A DIFFERENT LEVEL IN THE LEFT VS. RIGHT EAR ALL THE TIME? OR SHOULD I JUST KEEP IT AT ONE LEVEL IN BOTH EARS NO MATTER WHAT?

Yes, it would be better to setup the lowest audible volume for every ear separately.

Q: YOU MENTIONED SETTING THE LEVEL OF THE WHITE/PINK NOISE TO BE JUST BELOW THE TINNITUS, BUT WHAT IF THAT'S SO LOW YOU CAN'T EVEN HEAR IT... BASICALLY THE WHOLE DAY? BECAUSE I TYPICALLY DON'T HEAR MY TINNITUS DURING THE DAY, JUST AT NIGHT, THE WHITE/PINK NOISE WILL BE UNNOTICEABLE FOR ALMOST THE FULL 8 HOURS.

Pink noise must be at lowest audible level. It means tinnitus MUST be many times louder than pink noise. It is ok, if you listen to it just barely. You brain is perceiving it unconsciously.

I KNOW IN YOUR VIDEO YOU SAY TO USE OPEN HEADPHONES (THIS IS THE NAME FOR HEADPHONES THAT ENABLE YOU TO HEAR YOUR ENVIRONMENT AS WELL AS HEADPHONE SOUND (ALTHOUGH YOU COULD EASILY HEAR YOU'RE SURROUNDING WITH NORMAL HEADPHONES IF PINK NOISE IS AT LOW VOLUME.) I HAVE A PAIR THAT I USED FOR MIXING MUSIC AT

HOME. WHY IS THE QUALITY OF HEADPHONES AN ISSUE IF YOU'RE ONLY LISTENING TO PINK NOISE AT A MUCH LOWER VOLUME THAN TINNITUS?
The device needs to play all frequencies correctly on low volume.

Q: COULD I USE 'INSIDE EAR' WIRELESS HEADPHONES FOR MORE CONVENIENCE AND MANOEUVRABILITY WITH MY MP3 PLAYER?
Wireless not, as Bluetooth is radiation and you need to listen to pink noise sound 8 hours a day.

Q: CAN I DO SOME OF THE TRT IN BED WHILST ASLEEP, USING HIFI SPEAKERS TO PLAY THE PINK NOISE AT A MUCH LOWER VOLUME THAN TINNITUS? OR IS THE BRAIN NOT RECEPTIVE TO TREATMENT WHEN I AM ASLEEP/ DOES THE BRAIN STILL LISTEN TO THE SOUND WHEN I'M ASLEEP? I KNOW THE BRAIN IS ALWAYS ACTIVE BECAUSE WE CAN STILL BREATH AND WE CAN DREAM WHEN ASLEEP, AND OUR HEART STILL BEATS TO KEEP US ALIVE, ETC. OR DESPITE THIS, WILL THE BRAIN NOT LISTEN TO THE PINK NOISE BECAUSE IT'S ATTENTION IS ON THE DREAM SOUNDS OR NO SOUND AT ALL?
Please use sound enrichment instead of TRT during sleep.

Q: THANK YOU FOR YOUR BOOK, IT IS GOOD TO HAVE SOME HOPEFUL INFORMATION ABOUT THIS THING. I HAVE HAD TINNITUS FOR 3 MONTHS NOW. IS IT TOO SOON TO START TRT?
If you visit your ENT specialist and he didn't find any objective reason, you can start now.

Q: I ONLY HAVE IT IN THE RIGHT EAR. DOES THAT CHANGE ANYTHING ABOUT THE THERAPY, DO YOU THINK? A: THERAPY IS THE SAME.
Therapy is the same.

Q: DO YOU KNOW OF TRT EXPERTS IN ZURICH, OR AT LEAST, SWITZERLAND?
Unfortunately not, but you can ask here:
http://www.tinnitus-pjj.com/

Q: IS THE TINNITUS DIARY AVAILABLE FOR DOWNLOAD OR PURCHASE?
Yes, it is free for download, on my web.

Q: WHAT SUPPLEMENTS DO YOU RECOMMEND SUPPLEMENTS COULD HELP WITH TINNITUS?
Here are some, all have to be in organic quality.
- Oregano oil
- Omega 3 Lecithin
- Magnesium citrate chelate form
- Ferrum supplement

However more focus needs to be more on diet (no sugar, junk or chemicals in the food) as described in book before.n

Q: CAN I USE ANTIDEPRESSANTS? I READ THAT IT CAN INCREASE TINNITUS.
If your specialist prescribed you antidepressants because of tinnitus it can increase tinnitus. Read the side effects carefully and ask your specialist to prescribe you those with no tinnitus side effects. Also, treatment with antidepressants should be temporary and supplemented with psychotherapy. This needs to be always done with cooperation with your specialist (medical doctor). Also, ask your medical specialist to prescribe you the latest generation of antidepressants as some antidepressants from the past can increase tinnitus.

Q: CAN I GO TO A DENTIST WITH TINNITUS?
Yes you can, even if you have hyperacusis, just follow these steps:

1. During drilling, ask the dentist to stop every 10 seconds for 10 seconds before continuing. This way, you can withstand drilling even if you have tinnitus from acoustic trauma or hyperacusis.
2. Ask the dentist to use a rubber membrane in your mouth to prevent swallowing toxic waste from drilling (e.g., mercury) that can irritate your nervous system and increase tinnitus.

3. Use composite fillings instead of amalgam ones.

Tinnitus Success Story of George M.:

This is an example of how stress and amalgam fillings can lead to tinnitus. Half a year before developing tinnitus, George experienced stress during his divorce. Later, we discovered that he had suppressed anger that he had not expressed during the divorce. This inward anger was manifested through clenched jaws, which was confirmed during a physiotherapy examination. He also brushed his teeth more frequently due to the increased tension in his jaws, which led to brushing the amalgam fillings as well. Since amalgam contains heavy metals, his nervous system was irritated, resulting in tinnitus. During our consultations, we worked on raising his awareness and expressing his inner anger. He also gradually replaced his amalgam fillings with composite ones. Gradually, as he and his ex-partner spoke openly, his jaws relaxed, and his tinnitus changed to a pleasant pink noise that weakened to a level that no longer bothered him.

This example shows how stress can lead to tinnitus. It's also worth noting that dentists have the highest percentage of workers suffering from tinnitus. While I used to believe that this was caused by the drilling sound, I now know that amalgam fumes that dentists breathe daily can also be responsible for their tinnitus. As I have mentioned many times before, my cure involved a combination of several factors, and the amalgam problem was one of them.

Q: CAN I TRAVEL BY PLANE WITH TINNITUS?
Yes, here are five tips to help ensure your safety during your flight:
1. Wear earplugs in the airport until you are seated on the airplane to reduce exposure to loud engine noises.
2. Try to secure a seat at the front or back of the airplane (depending on the aircraft's make) to avoid sitting close to

the wings where the engines are located.
3. Chew gum during the flight to help alleviate ear discomfort and pressure changes.
4. If the sound level in the airplane is lower than 65 dB, you may use your TRT device. If it's higher, noise-canceling headphones with soothing music can be used instead. If the sound level exceeds 75 dB, it's best to wear earplugs.
5. The same guidelines apply to helicopters. Ask the pilot to reduce the volume on your intercom if necessary.

By following these tips, you can have a safer and more comfortable flight experience.

CONCLUSION

""Feelings of helplessness, immobility, and freezing. If hyperarousal is the nervous system's accelerator, a sense of overwhelming helplessness is its brake. The helplessness that is experienced at such times is not the ordinary sense of helplessness that can affect anyone from time to time. It is the sense of being collapsed, immobilised, and utterly helpless. It is not a perception, belief, or a trick of the imagination. It is real."

Peter Levine

I hope that the book has given you clear understanding how to get tinnitus relief step-by-step. You should know and believe that there are plenty of people who have cured tinnitus and if you follow TRT and solve the underlying psychological issues, you can end your tinnitus too. TRT therapy does not focus on the problem in the ear (such as narrowed coils, inflammation, cervical spine problems that affect nerve in the ear, impaired hearing, calcification, etc.), but instead on the real problem – unconscious filters in our brain. But not only did TRT cure my tinnitus as I explained before. I had to made few bigger changes in my life to get complete relief.

What changed in my life and what had the effect my cure?
- I got divorced. I refused to listen to constant complaints.
- I sold my company to my partner. I worked in the company after normal work and it was common for me to work 16

hours a day. After I sold the company, I relaxed more.
- I found a new job that makes me more satisfied.
- I attended seminars held by Dan Millman and Brandon Bays. All, in a few years, changed my life and solved a lot of problems that caused me stress. I also learned to cry from time to time. I learned a lot about myself and it helped me a lot in all aspects of life.
- And last, but not least, what is most important: tinnitus in my world no longer exists :)

What else I do after this experience?
- I'm going back to the cinema – with earplugs.
- I'm going to parties in the clubs – with earplugs.
- I go to concerts – with earplugs.
- When an ambulance approaches, or a police car, I cover my ears with hands until it passes.
- When seeing a dentist, I always make one tooth and if needed, next teeth I will go for repair after 2 weeks, to minimize long strong sound. If you need to go to the dentist, request laser instead of a mechanical drill. Also ask the dentist, if he or she can drill for 30 seconds and then pause for 30 seconds.
- For dental hygiene, I will ask for the removal of the teeth mechanically, without ultrasound.
- In the underground/subway, at motor races I use earplugs.
- On New Year's Eve, I take the strongest earplugs and spend it outside the big city with my dog :).
- And a critical point: when I applaud, or am in an environment where I expect applause, I also use earplugs. On one occasion, during a Ludovico Einaudi concert, I was without earplugs the whole time and it was ok. But at the end there was applause for ten minutes, and this caused me to be sensitive to any sound for two weeks (fortunately I knew what to do and I was fit again in short time).
- I started playing a electric violin, which allows me to adjust the volume.

- I exercise more, running, dancing (I have half earplugs for dance training). For yoga, take great care to get it right. During treatment, I would not recommend yoga as it can worsen your tinnitus.
- I found a psychosomatic reason – my tinnitus was related to the fact that I was constantly feeling regret and holding back the sadness and anger. So now if someone is not nice to me, I tell him and if he continues, I stop seeing him. If there is something sad, I cry.
- I still have my earplugs and I am not ashamed to use them in public.
- When I'm accidentally exposed to a stronger sound, I'll go 2 days without music.
- I avoid silence. Complete silence is unnatural to the human brain. We have been evolving for thousands of years, and the silence we have at night is unnatural. For example, before now, windows were made with wood and those wood windows caused natural sound to come into the rooms, but now, new technology such as plastic windows, are replacing the old wood windows and the result is that when a new technology window is closed, you cannot hear anything from the outside.
- When you look at any kind of documentary about nature, everything in nature is silent when the predator approaches. That's why the brain is very active in silence – much more than when there is a bit of background noise (for example, wind, or distant voices from the street).
- During a year of helping others, I realized another useful thing: it is best to set the volume of the pink or white noise in the morning in a quiet room. And if you follow the rule that the volume of pink or white noise is lower that volume of your tinnitus, you can track your progress. You will see whether your tinnitus is stronger or weaker than yesterday. You can then go through the day before and find out when your tinnitus gets weaker and when it gets stronger. Then you can then make appropriate changes to

your lifestyle, as certain aspects of your diet, exercise, or certain relationships are increasing your tinnitus, while other things in your life make it better. Together with TRT therapy, it will drop to the level you will stop perceiving it, the way it was with me. Another good thing about this accurate measurement is that you do not have to watch tinnitus levels ~~over~~ during the day. You will have information from the next morning and you will not need to monitor your tinnitus and be worried about it.

That's everything. If you have questions, you can visit my site www.icuredmytinnitus.com, or send me an email. I remember how I wrote about 50 questions to Dr. Jastreboff during half a year, and he responded patiently to all of them. It helped me so much and it gave me peace. Don't be alone with your problem.

And remember: many people, including myself, have cured their tinnitus. You can do it too.

LAST WORDS BY AUTHOR

Dear reader,

I would like to personally thank you for choosing my book *I cured my Tinnitus*. I know that trusting someone is not easy and I appreciate the trust you gave me. I wrote the book to make tinnitus cure possible for others. I want everybody to know that they don't need to suffer so badly and for so long as I did.

The book has been updated over the years to help others as much as possible. For many readers, my book has become an important part of their cure and that is the biggest reward for me.

All that I have written here and suggested, need to be followed and done properly. My wish is that my story, book and consultations help to cure tinnitus for as many people as possible. If you need anything to clarify, add or explain, please write to me and I will reply, doing my best to help you.

My address is pstudenik@hotmail.com.

Get well soon,
Peter Studenik MS
#1 Amazon best-selling author of I cured my Tinnitus

NOTE TO READERS

This book represents my own knowledge and experience. Although I believe that it will inspire you to find a way to cure your tinnitus and hyperacusis, keep in mind that I am not a doctor. The contents of this book and my website, such as text, graphics, images, and other material contained on the website ("content"), are for informational purposes only and do not constitute medical advice; the Content is not intended to be a substitute for professional medical advice, diagnosis, or treatment. Always seek the advice of a physician or other qualified health provider with any questions you may have regarding a medical condition. Never disregard professional medical advice or delay in seeking it because of something you have read in this book or on my website.

Neither the publisher nor I shall be responsible for any damage resulting directly or indirectly from the information contained in this book.

If you decide to follow my suggestions and recommendations, be sure that your doctor(s) has confirmed that you don't have a physiological cause of tinnitus. The best would be, if you can find a doctor who is familiar with TRT therapy and is an expert in psychosomatics who can supervise you during therapy.

I wish you the best and believe that you will find your way to cure your tinnitus, as I did.

Please stay in touch and find fresh information here:

Web: www.icuredmytinnitus.com
Blog and FAQs www.icuredmytinnitus.com/faq
Facebook: www.facebook.com/icuredmytinnitus/
YouTube: https://cutt.ly/0kwuxKK

On Facebook pages, I regularly answer questions sent by my

clients. If you want to see all new questions and answers, you can subscribe Facebook or Youtube. Also, do not hesitate to contact me in case you need help.

ACKNOWLEDGMENTS

Thank you to Dr. Pawel Jastreboff, Dr. Susan Velda, Alice Miller, Dr. Peter A. Levine PhD., Dr. Vladimir Vogeltanz, Dr. Bessel van der Kolk, Dan Millman and Michaela Lipkova for their support, patience, and especially for being healthy. Thanx go also to Jeff Bussell and David Luster for their help and corrections in English version.

Printed in Great Britain
by Amazon